Study Guide for
Understanding
Nursing Research

SECOND EDITION

Nancy Burns, *PhD, RN, FAAN*
Jenkins Garrett Professor
School of Nursing
University of Texas at Arlington
Arlington, Texas

Susan K. Grove, *PhD, RN, CS, ANP, GNP*
Professor of Nursing
Assistant Dean, Graduate Nursing Program
School of Nursing
University of Texas at Arlington
Arlington, Texas

W.B. SAUNDERS COMPANY
A Division of Harcourt Brace & Company
Philadelphia   London   Toronto   Montreal   Sydney   Tokyo

W.B. SAUNDERS COMPANY

A Division of Harcourt Brace & Company

The Curtis Center
Independence Square West
Philadelphia, PA 19106

Study Guide for
UNDERSTANDING NURSING RESEARCH, 2/e   ISBN 0–7216–8108–5

Printed in the United States of America.

Last digit is the print number: 9 8 7 6 5 4 3 2 1

PREFACE

The amount of knowledge generated through research is rapidly escalating in nursing. This knowledge is critical to the promotion of quality, cost effective nursing care. As a baccalaureate-prepared nurse, you will be encouraged to read and use research findings to develop protocols and policies for practice. We recognize that learning research terminology and reading and critiquing research reports are complex and sometimes overwhelming activities. Thus, we have developed this study guide to assist you in clarifying, comprehending, analyzing, synthesizing, and applying the content presented in your textbook, *Understanding Nursing Research,* 2nd edition. This edition of your study guide has been reorganized according to the steps of the research process, with the chapter on problem and purpose prior to the review of literature chapter. The text and the study guide include additional information on qualitative research and provide an introduction to outcomes research. This second edition of the study guide provides exercises that address the revised content on literature review, ethics, and measurement.

Your study guide is organized into thirteen chapters, which correspond to the chapters of your textbook. In each chapter of your study guide you will encounter learning exercises that require various levels of critical thinking skills. These exercises are organized using the following headings: Relevant Terms, Key Ideas, Making Connections, Puzzles, Exercises in Critique, and Going Beyond. In some exercises, you will define relevant terms or identify key ideas. In other exercises, you will be demonstrating comprehension of the research process by connecting one idea to another. Some exercises are puzzles that will make learning research fun. In the most complex exercises, you will apply your new research knowledge by conducting critiques of published studies.

After completing the exercises for each chapter, you will be able to review the answers in Appendix A and assess your understanding of the content. Based on your correct and incorrect responses, you will be able to focus your study to improve your knowledge of each chapter's content.

Since your learning is enhanced by exposure to a variety of visual and writing exercises, we have included a computer disk in the back of your study guide. This disk includes multiple choice review questions to promote your understanding and application of research knowledge. Completing the exercises in the study guide and the computer disk provides you with a background for analyzing and synthesizing the findings from research reports for application in practice.

INTRODUCTION

This *Study Guide* was developed to accompany the textbook, *Understanding Nursing Research,* 2nd edition. The exercises in this guide were designed to assist you in comprehending the content in your textbook, conducting critiques of nursing studies, and using research findings in practice. You need to read each chapter in your text before completing the chapters in this guide. Scan the entire chapter to get an overall view of the content. Then reread the chapter with the intent of increasing your comprehension of each section. As you examine each section, pay careful attention to the terms that are defined. Underline or highlight definitions of terms in the text. If the meaning of a term is not clear to you, look up its definition in the glossary at the back of the book or in a dictionary. Highlight key ideas in each section. Examine tables and figures as they are referred to in the text. Mark sections you do not feel you sufficiently understand. Reread these sections one sentence at a time to increase your understanding. Jot down questions to ask your instructor in class or privately.

After carefully reading a chapter in the text, use the study guide to further enhance your understanding. Each chapter in the study guide corresponds to its related chapter in your textbook. There are six main sections to each study guide chapter: Relevant Terms, Key Ideas, Making Connections, Puzzles, Exercises in Critique, and Going Beyond.

Relevant Terms

Relevant Terms have been identified for each chapter to assist you in becoming familiar with essential terminology for understanding the research process. Knowing these terms before you attend a class lecture on the content will give you an edge in grasping the lecture content and doing well on course exams. As you read the text, do not skip over terms in the chapter that are unfamiliar to you. Get in the habit of marking unfamiliar words as you read and looking up their definitions in the glossary at the end of the text.

Key Ideas

This section of the study guide identifies important information in each chapter for you. The fill-in-the-blank form of questions includes both short- and long-answer format and will assist you in identifying essential chapter content that you might have missed. You may need to refer to specific sections of the text to complete some of the questions.

Making Connections

The Making Connections exercises promote linking significant ideas together to facilitate the comprehension, analysis, and synthesis of content related to the research process. Matching questions are frequently used to assist you in performing these critical thinking skills.

Puzzles

The Puzzles section is designed for having fun while learning the research process. The **Word Scramble** contains important ideas expressed in the chapter, but the letters in each word have been scrambled. For example, "study" might be scrambled to read "tysud." You will need to unscramble the words to get the message. The **Secret Message** contains another important idea expressed in the chapter. To decipher the message, you must identify the code used and decode the message. For example, one secret message might have been coded by moving each letter of the alphabet down three letters. In this case, A = D, B = E, C = F, etc. Once you identify a few letters, you have clues you can use to guess at other letters in words. You may find it easier to start with the short words. Also, remember that the most commonly used letter in our language is e. The **Crossword Puzzles** were developed to help you increase your familiarity with the terms used in the chapter.

Exercises in Critique

Critique exercises are provided to give you experience in critiquing published studies. In some cases, brief quotes are provided with questions addressing information specific to the chapter content. The critique exercises focus on the three published studies that are provided in Appendix B of this study guide. On completing the study guide, you can incorporate the critique information you have developed to perform an overall critique of these three studies. In addition, you can take the knowledge you have learned and apply it in the critique of other published studies.

Going Beyond

Exercises have been included that provide suggestions for further study. You might use these activities to test your new knowledge. If the content of a particular chapter interests you, this section might direct you in learning more about that step of the research process.

Answers

The answers to all *Study Guide* questions are provided in **Appendix A** in the back of the *Study Guide*. However, we would recommend that you not refer to these answers except to check your own responses to the questions. You will learn more by reading the textbook and searching for the answers on your own.

Published Studies

Reprints of three published studies are provided in **Appendix B.** These studies are referred to in many of the study questions throughout the *Study Guide*.

CONTENTS

CHAPTER 1
DISCOVERING NURSING RESEARCH

⌘ INTRODUCTION

Read Chapter 1 and then complete the following exercises. These exercises will assist you in learning relevant terms and identifying the types of research conducted in nursing. The answers to these exercises are in Appendix A under Chapter 1.

⌘ RELEVANT TERMS

♦ **Directions:** Match each term below with its correct definition.

a. authority
b. deductive reasoning
c. explanation
d. inductive reasoning
e. intuition
f. knowledge
g. nursing research
h. outcomes research
i. personal experience
j. prediction
k. qualitative research
l. quantitative research
m. reasoning
n. research
o. scientific methods

Definitions

_____ 1. Information acquired in a variety of ways that is expected to be an accurate reflection of reality.
_____ 2. Scientific process that validates and refines existing knowledge and generates new knowledge that directly and indirectly influences nursing practice.
_____ 3. Person with expertise and power who is able to influence the opinion of others.
_____ 4. Reasoning from the specific to the general.
_____ 5. Gaining knowledge by being personally involved in an event, situation, or circumstance.
_____ 6. Formal, objective, systematic research process to describe, test relationships among, or examine cause-and-effect interactions among variables.

_____ 7. Reasoning from the general to the specific or from a general premise to a particular situation.

_____ 8. Procedures that scientists have used, currently use, or may use in the future to pursue knowledge.

_____ 9. Insight or understanding of a situation or event as a whole that usually cannot be explained logically.

_____ 10. Diligent, systematic inquiry to validate and refine existing knowledge and generate new knowledge.

_____ 11. Systematic, subjective research approach used to describe life experiences and give them meaning.

_____ 12. Knowledge generated from research that clarifies relationships among variables and identifies the reasons why certain events occur.

_____ 13. An important scientific methodology that was developed to examine the end results of patient care.

_____ 14. Type of thinking that involves processing and organizing ideas in order to reach conclusions.

_____ 15. Knowledge generated from research that enables one to estimate the probability of a specific outcome in a given situation.

⌘ KEY IDEAS

♦ **Directions:** The knowledge generated through research is essential to provide a scientific basis for **description, explanation, prediction,** and **control** of nursing practice. Write a definition and provide an example of these four terms.

1. Description: _____

_____

_____

Example: _____

2. Explanation: _____

_____

_____

Example: _____

3. Prediction: _____

_____

_____

Example: _____

4. Control: _____

_____

_____

Example: _____

Historical Events Influencing Nursing Research

♦ **Directions:** Fill in the blanks in this section with the appropriate word(s) or numbers.

1. _____ is considered the first nurse researcher.

2. The journal *Nursing Research* was first published in _____.

3. The American Nurses Association (ANA) Commission on Nursing Research established the _____ in 1972.

4. Many national and international _____ conferences have been sponsored by Sigma Theta Tau, the international honor society for nursing since 1970.

5. The nursing research journal first published in 1978 is _____

_____.

6. The research journal first published in 1979 is _____

_____.

7. Identify three other journals that were first published in 1987 or 1988.

   a. _____

   b. _____

   c. _____

8. _____ was the project directed by Horsley to promote the use of research findings in practice; the project results were published in 1982–1983.

9. The *Annual Review of Nursing Research* includes _____

_____

_____

10. The National Center for Nursing Research (NCNR) was established in _____ by the National Institutes of Health.

11. The NCNR is now called the _____.

12. The purpose of the National Institute for Nursing research (NINR) is

   _____, _____, and

   _____ regarding basic clinical nursing research.

13. Identify four research priorities of the NINR for 1995–1999.

   a. _____

   b. _____

   c. _____

   d. _____

14. The focus of the 1980s and 1990s is the conduct of _____ research.

15. _____ was established in

   1989 to facilitate the conduct of outcomes research and the communication of the

   findings to health care practitioners.

16. The conduct of numerous, high-quality studies is essential for the development of a

   _____ knowledge base for nursing practice.

Acquiring Knowledge in Nursing

♦ **Directions:** Fill in the blanks with the appropriate responses.

1. List seven ways to acquire knowledge in nursing and provide an example of each.

   a. _____

   b. _____

   c. _____

   d. _____

   e. _____

   f. _____

   g. _____

2. Benner's (1984) book *From novice to expert: Excellence and power in clinical practice*
   describes the importance of _____ in
   acquiring nursing knowledge.

3. Identify Benner's five levels of experience in the development of clinical knowledge and expertise.

   a. _____   d. _____

   b. _____   e. _____

   c. _____

4. Nursing has _____ knowledge from other disciplines such as medicine, physiology, and sociology.

5. _____ knowledge provides a scientific basis for description, explanation, prediction, and control of nursing practice.

6. "Gut feeling" or "hunch" is an example of _____ that nurses have found useful in identifying serious patient problems.

7. _____ are knowledge based on customs and past trends, such as providing hospitalized patients a bath every morning.

8. New graduates sometimes enter internships provided by clinical agencies and are guided, supported, and educated by experienced nurses. This is an example of a _____

   _____.

9. In the internship, new graduates are encouraged to _____, or imitate the behaviors of expert nurses.

10. Two types of logical reasoning are _____ and

    _____.

11. What type of reasoning is used in the following example? _____
    Human beings experience pain.
    Babies are human beings.
    Therefore, babies experience pain.

12. Identify the types of research that are essential for the generation of knowledge for nursing practice: _____, _____,

    and _____.

13. What type of research is conducted to examine the cost-effectiveness of health care?

    _____ _____

14. Identify five interventions that you use frequently in your nursing practice. Next to each intervention, identify the knowledge base for that intervention.

Intervention	_Knowledge Base_
a. _____	_____
b. _____	_____
c. _____	_____
d. _____	_____
e. _____	_____

15. What type of knowledge is the basis for the majority of your interventions in clinical practice? _____

16. Identify four important outcomes that might be examined with outcomes research.

   a. _____

   b. _____

   c. _____

   d. _____

⌘ MAKING CONNECTIONS

Types of Research Methods

♦ **Directions:** Match the following research methods with the specific types of research.

   a. qualitative research method
   b. quantitative research method

____ 1. correlational research
____ 2. descriptive research
____ 3. ethnographic research
____ 4. experimental research
____ 5. grounded theory research
____ 6. historical research
____ 7. phenomenological research
____ 8. quasi-experimental research

Nurses' Educational Preparation

♦ **Directions:** Match the levels of nurses' educational preparation with the research activities for which each group of nurses is primarily responsible according to the guidelines of the American Nurses Association (ANA).

Nurses' Educational Preparation

    a. associate degree
    b. baccalaureate degree
    c. master's degree

    d. doctoral degree (PhD or DNS)
    e. post-doctorate

Research Activities

_____ 1. Uses research findings in practice with supervision.
_____ 2. Develops and coordinates funded research programs.
_____ 3. Critiques studies.
_____ 4. Develops nursing knowledge through research and theory development.
_____ 5. Uses research findings in practice.
_____ 6. Collaborates in conducting research projects.
_____ 7. Conducts funded independent research projects.

⌘ PUZZLES

Word Scramble

♦ **Directions:** Unscramble the words in the following sentences to determine their meaning.

1. Tobh tiqutaantive nad aliqutaivet sereacrh era esenstial to evledpo singnur ledknegow.

2. Searerch nowkdegle si deende to trconol tcosuome in urinngs actripce.

⌘ EXERCISES IN CRITIQUE

♦ **Directions:** Locate the research articles in Appendix B. Review the titles and abstracts of these three articles. Identify the type of research conducted in each study.

    a. outcomes research method
    b. qualitative research method
    c. quantitative research method

_____ 1. Bruce & Grove (1994)
_____ 2. Lewis, Nichols, Mackey, Fadol, Sloane, Villagomez, & Liehr (1997)
_____ 3. Berg, Dunbar-Jacob, & Sereika (1997)

♦ **Directions:** Review the educational credentials of the authors of the three research articles in Appendix B.

1. Do Berg *et al.* (1997) have the educational preparation to conduct their study? Explain.

2. Do Lewis *et al.* (1997) have the educational preparation to conduct their study? Explain.

3. Do Bruce & Grove (1994) have the educational preparation to conduct their study? Explain.

⌘ GOING BEYOND

1. Locate the most recent copy of the *Applied Nursing Research* or *Nursing Research* journal. Identify the research method (qualitative, quantitative, or outcomes) used in each study. Provide a rationale for your answer. Ask your instructor to verify your answers.

2. Find a faculty member who is conducting research. Ask if you can participate in the collection of data for this project. Can this faculty member serve as your mentor as you learn the research process?

CHAPTER 2
INTRODUCTION TO THE
QUANTITATIVE RESEARCH
PROCESS

⌘ INTRODUCTION

Read Chapter 2 and then complete the following exercises. These exercises will assist you in learning the steps of the quantitative research process, identifying the different types of quantitative research (descriptive, correlational, quasi-experimental, and experimental), and reading research reports. The answers to these exercises are in Appendix A under Chapter 2.

⌘ RELEVANT TERMS

♦ **Directions:** Match each term below with its correct definition.

a. abstract	k. nursing process
b. applied research	l. pilot study
c. assumption	m. problem-solving process
d. basic research	n. quantitative research process
e. control	o. reading research reports
f. design	p. research report
g. framework	q. rigor
h. generalization	r. sampling
i. methodological limitations	s. setting
j. methods section	t. theoretical limitations

Definitions

_____ 1. Formal, objective, systematic process to describe and test relationships and to examine cause-and-effect interactions among variables.

_____ 2. Location for conducting research that can be natural, partially controlled, or highly controlled.

_____ 3. Scientific investigations conducted to generate knowledge that will directly influence clinical practice.

_____ 4. Imposing of rules by the researcher to decrease the possibility of error and increase the probability that the study's findings are an accurate reflection of reality.

_____ 5. Process of selecting a group of people, events, behaviors, or other elements that are representative of the population being studied.

_____ 6. Scientific investigations for the pursuit of "knowledge for knowledge's sake" or for the pleasure of learning.

_____ 7. Process used to direct patient care that involves assessment, diagnosis, planning, implementation, evaluation, and modification.

_____ 8. Striving for excellence in research through the use of discipline, scrupulous adherence to detail, and strict accuracy.

_____ 9. Extension of the implications of the findings from the sample that was studied to the larger population.

_____ 10. Smaller version of a proposed study conducted to develop and/or refine the methodology, such as the treatment, instruments, or data collection process, to be used in the larger study.

_____ 11. Process that involves systematic identification of a problem, determination of goals, identification of possible approaches to achieve goals, implementation of the approaches, and evaluation of goal achievement.

_____ 12. Statements that are taken for granted or are considered true even though they have not been scientifically tested.

_____ 13. The limitations that restrict the abstract generalization of the findings and are reflected in the study framework and the conceptual and operational definitions of the variables.

_____ 14. A clear, concise summary of a study that usually is placed at the beginning of a study and is about 100–125 words.

_____ 15. Involves skills of skimming, comprehending, and analyzing content from research reports.

_____ 16. Report summarizing the major elements of a study and identifying the contributions of that study to nursing knowledge.

_____ 17. The section of the research report that describes how the study was conducted and usually includes the design, sample, setting, methods of measurement, and data collection process.

_____ 18. Limitations that decrease the credibility of the findings and restrict the population to which the findings can be generalized.

_____ 19. The abstract, theoretical basis for a study that enables the researcher to link the findings to nursing's body of knowledge.

_____ 20. Blueprint for the conduct of a study that maximizes control over factors that could interfere with the study's desired outcome.

⌘ KEY IDEAS

Control in Quantitative Research

◆ **Directions:** Fill in the blanks with the appropriate word(s).

1. An experimental study is conducted in a _____ setting.

2. Extraneous variables need to be controlled in _____ and
   _____ types of quantitative research to ensure that the findings
   are an accurate reflection of reality.

3. _____ or _____ studies are usually
   uncontrolled by the researcher and are conducted in natural settings.

4. _____ studies require random selection of the sample.

5. Frequently a _____ sampling method is used in descriptive and
   correlational studies. However, a _____ sampling method might
   also be used.

6. A subject's home is an example of a _____ setting.

7. Laboratories and research centers are examples of _____
   settings.

8. Researcher control is greatest in _____ quantitative research.

9. Hospital units are _____ settings that allow the researcher to
   control some of the extraneous variables.

10. _____ research is conducted to determine the effect of a
    treatment but often involves less control than experimental research.

Steps of the Research Process

◆ **Directions:** Fill in the blanks in this section with the appropriate word(s).

1. The research process is similar to the _____ and the
   _____ processes.

2. The nursing diagnosis step of the nursing process is similar to the

_____ and _____ steps of the research

process.

3. The plan of the nursing process is similar to the _____ section

of the research process.

4. The evaluation and modification steps of the nursing process are similar to the

_____ and _____ steps of the

problem-solving process. However, the last steps of the research process,

_____ ,

_____ ,

and_____ ,

are quite different.

5. List the steps of the quantitative research process in their order of occurrence.

Step 1   _____

Step 2   _____

Step 3   _____

Step 4   _____

Step 5   _____

Step 6   _____

Step 7   _____

Step 8   _____

Step 9   _____

Step 10   _____

Step 11   _____

Step 12   _____

Step 13   _____

6. Assumptions are:_____

_____

7. Identify four common assumptions on which nursing studies have been based.

    a. _____

    b. _____

    c. _____

    d. _____

8. The two types of limitations that might exist in a study are _____

   and _____.

9. Identify five examples of limitations that you might find in published studies.

    a. _____

    b. _____

    c. _____

    d. _____

    e. _____

10. A pilot study is: _____

   _____

11. Identify five reasons for conducting a pilot study.

    a. _____

    b. _____

    c. _____

    d. _____

    e. _____

Reading Research Reports

1. The most common sources for nursing research reports are professional journals. Identify three nursing research journals.

    a. _____

    b. _____

    c. _____

2. Identify three clinical journals in which research reports compose 50% or more of the journal content.

    a. _____

    b. _____

    c. _____

3. Identify the four major sections of a research report.

    a. _____   c. _____

    b. _____   d. _____

4. The methods section of a research report describes how a study was conducted and usually includes:

    a. _____   d. _____

    b. _____   e. _____

    c. _____

5. The discussion section ties the other sections of the research report together and gives them meaning. This section includes:

    a. _____

    b. _____

    c. _____

    d. _____

    e. _____

6. In which section of a research report are the problem and purpose often identified?

    _____

7. The reference list at the end of the article includes all the _____ and _____ that provide a basis for this study and are cited in the article.

8. Reading a research report involves _____,

    _____, and _____ the content of the report.

9. In reading a research report, the _____ step involves identifying the steps of the research process.

10. In reading a research report, _____ involves determining the value of the report's content by determining the quality and completeness of the steps of the research process and examining logical links among these steps.

⌘ MAKING CONNECTIONS

Types of Quantitative Research

♦ **Directions:** Match the type of quantitative research listed below with the example study titles.

        a. descriptive research
        b. correlational research
        c. quasi-experimental research
        d. experimental research

_____ 1. Determining the effect of a relaxation technique on patients' post-operative pain and anxiety level.

_____ 2. Identifying the incidence of HIV in adolescents and young adults.

_____ 3. Examining the relationships among age, gender, knowledge of AIDS, and use of condoms in college students.

_____ 4. Describing the coping strategies of chronically ill men and women.

_____ 5. Determining the effects of position on sacral and heel pressures in hospitalized elderly patients.

_____ 6. Determining the effect of impaired physical mobility on skeletal muscle atrophy in laboratory rats.

_____ 7. Identifying current nursing practice for male and female nurses.

_____ 8. Examining the relationship among intensive care unit (ICU) stress, anxiety, and recovery rate for patients following cardiac surgery.

_____ 9. Examining the effects of a preadmission self-instruction program on patients' post-operative activity level, anxiety level, pain perception, length of hospital stay, and time returning to work.

_____ 10. Examining the effects of thermal applications on the abdominal temperature of laboratory dogs.

_____ 11. Examining the relationships among hardiness, depression, and coping in institutionalized elderly patients.

_____ 12. Determining the incidence of drug abuse in registered nurses in community and hospital settings.

_____ 13. Examining the effect of warm and cold applications on the resolution of IV infiltrations in hospitalized patients.

_____ 14. Determining the stress levels and desired support of family caregivers of elderly adults with Alzheimer's disease.

_____ 15. Examining the effectiveness of a breast cancer screening program for women residing in rural areas.

_____ 16. Comparing the age and coping skills of mothers pregnant with their first child in three ethnic groups (Caucasian, African American, and Hispanic).

_____ 17. Using age, nutritional intake, mobility level, weight, level of cognitive function, and serum albumin to predict the risk of pressure ulcers in hospitalized patients on a medical-surgical unit.

_____ 18. Describing the severity of fatigue and anxiety in individuals with chronic obstructive pulmonary disease.

_____ 19. Comparing and contrasting the health promotion and illness prevention behaviors of African American and Caucasian older adults.

_____ 20. Examining the relationships among the lipid values, blood pressure, weight, and stress levels of adolescents.

⌘ PUZZLES

Word Scramble

♦ **Directions:** Unscramble the words in the following sentences to determine their meaning.

1. Taquntiatiev sereacrh thodmes duclein cridpseitve, rrelacotiaonl,

   saiqu-perexienmtal, dna eperxmiealnt udiests.

2. Gorir dan rotconl ear pormtinta ni utitavieqtan chrearse.

Crossword Puzzle

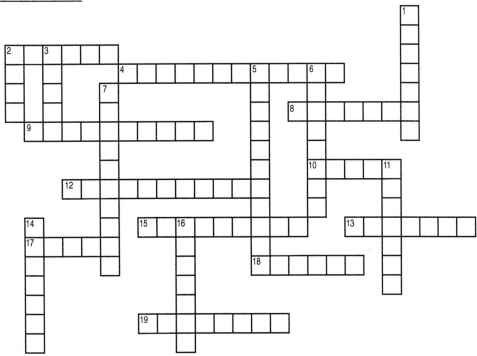

Across
2. study blueprint
4. research method
8. nursing concern
9. null ____
10. type of research that seeks knowledge for knowledge's sake
12. ____ of dependent variables in research
13. location of research
15. Crisis theory could be a study ____.
17. strict adherence to research plan
18. subjects comprise this
19. directs a study

Down
1. research finding
2. What is collected in a study?
3. research project
5. known truths
6. Study treatment is an independent ____.
7. What is reviewed prior to conducting a study?
11. Researchers ____ extraneous variables.
14. nursing ____ to direct nursing care
16. Practice-related studies are ____ research.

⌘ EXERCISES IN CRITIQUE

Type of Quantitative Research

♦ **Directions:** Read the research articles in Appendix B. Identify the type of quantitative research conducted in each study.

    a. descriptive research
    b. correlational research
    c. quasi-experimental research
    d. experimental research

_____   1. "An Evaluation of a Self-Management Program for Adults with Asthma" (Berg, *et al.,* 1997)
_____   2. "The Effect of Turning and Backrub on Mixed Venous Oxygen Saturation in critically ill patients" (Lewis, *et al.,* 1997)
_____   3. "The Effect of a Coronary Artery Risk Evaluation Program on Serum Lipid Values and Cardiovascular Risk Levels" (Bruce and Grove, 1994)

Type of Setting

♦ **Directions:** Identify the type of setting for each study.

    a. natural setting
    b. partially controlled setting
    c. highly controlled setting

_____   4. Berg, *et al.* (1997) study
_____   5. Lewis *et al.* (1997) study
_____   6. Bruce and Grove (1994) study

Type of Research Conducted

♦ **Directions:** Indicate the type of nursing research conducted.

    a. applied nursing research
    b. basic nursing research

_____   7. Berg, *et al.* (1997) study
_____   8. Lewis *et al.* (1997) study
_____   9. Bruce and Grove (1994) study

CHAPTER 3
RESEARCH PROBLEMS,
PURPOSES, AND HYPOTHESES

⌘ INTRODUCTION

Read Chapter 3 and then complete the following exercises. These exercises will assist you in critiquing problems, purposes, objectives, questions, hypotheses, and variables in published studies. The answers to these exercises are in Appendix A under Chapter 3.

⌘ RELEVANT TERMS

♦ **Directions:** Match each term below with its correct definition.

a. conceptual definition of variable   g. operational definition of variable
b. demographic variable   h. research problem
c. dependent variable   i. research purpose
d. hypothesis   j. research topic
e. independent variable   k. research question
f. landmark study

Definitions

____ 1. Major, significant study generating knowledge that influences a discipline and sometimes society.
____ 2. Clear, concise statement of the specific goal or aim of the study that is generated from the problem.
____ 3. Situation in need of solution, improvement, or alteration or a discrepancy between the way things are and the way they ought to be.
____ 4. Description of how variables will be measured or manipulated in a study.

_____ 5. Concise interrogative statement developed to direct a study; focuses on description of variables, examination of relationship among variables, and determination of differences between two or more groups.

_____ 6. Concept or broad problem area that provides the basis for generating numerous research problems.

_____ 7. The treatment or experimental activity that is manipulated or varied by the researcher to create an effect on the dependent variable.

_____ 8. Formal statement of the expected relationship among or expected outcome of two or more variables in a specified population.

_____ 9. Definition that provides a variable or concept with connotative (abstract, comprehensive, theoretical) meaning; established through concept analysis, concept derivation, or concept synthesis.

_____ 10. The response, behavior, or outcome that is predicted or explained in research; changes in this variable are presumed to be caused by the independent variable.

_____ 11. Characteristics or attributes of subjects that are collected to describe the sample.

Types of Hypotheses

♦ **Directions:** Match each type of hypothesis with the correct definition.

a. associative hypothesis   e. nondirectional hypothesis
b. causal hypothesis   f. null hypothesis
c. complex hypothesis   g. research hypothesis
d. directional hypothesis   h. simple hypothesis

Definitions

_____ 1. Hypothesis stating the relationship (associative or causal) between two variables.

_____ 2. Alternative hypothesis to the null hypothesis; states that a relationship exists between two or more variables.

_____ 3. Hypothesis stating a relationship in which an independent variable is thought to cause or determine the presence of a dependent variable.

_____ 4. Hypothesis that states that a relationship exists but does not predict the exact nature of the relationship.

_____ 5. Hypothesis predicting the relationships (associative or causal) among three or more variables.

_____ 6. Hypothesis stating a relationship in which variables or concepts that occur or exist together in the real world are identified; thus, when one variable changes, the other variable changes.

_____ 7. Hypothesis stating the specific nature of the interaction or relationship between two or more variables.

_____ 8. Hypothesis stating that no relationship exists between the variables being studied.

Variables

◆ **Directions:** Match each term with the appropriate example.

a. conceptual definition
b. demographic variable
c. dependent variable

d. extraneous variable
e. independent variable
f. operational definition

Definitions

_____ 1. Pain is a physiologic and psychologic response to a stimulus that occurs whenever and to the degree that a patient says it does.

_____ 2. Variables that exist in all studies and can affect the measurement of study variables and the relationships among these variables, such as changes in the environment, interaction with other people, or the health status of a patient.

_____ 3. The patient's pain will be measured with a visual analog scale and the Perception of Pain Likert Scale.

_____ 4. The variables of heart rate, blood pressure, and respiratory rate that are measured after the completion of an exercise program.

_____ 5. Treatment of ambulating a patient every 2–4 hours.

_____ 6. Variables such as age, gender, and ethnic origin measured to describe the sample.

⌘ KEY IDEAS

Research Problem and Purpose

◆ **Directions:** Fill in the blanks with the correct responses.

1. A clearly stated research purpose includes:

   a. _____

   b. _____

   c. _____

2. Research problems and purposes are significant if they have the potential to generate and refine relevant knowledge that:

   a. _____

   b. _____

   c. _____

   d. _____

3. Identify two organizations or agencies that have developed lists of research priorities relevant to nursing:

    a. _____

    b. _____

4. The feasibility of a research problem and purpose is determined by examining:

    a. _____

    b. _____

    c. _____

    d. _____

5. Two ways to determine research expertise is by examining the _____ preparation and _____ experience of the researchers.

6. _____, _____, and _____ evolve from the purpose and provide direction for the remaining steps of the research process.

⌘ EXERCISES IN CRITIQUE

Berg, *et al.* Study

♦ **Directions:** Review the Berg *et al.* (1997) article in Appendix B and answer the following questions.

1. State the problem addressed in this study.

2. State the purpose of this study.

3. Are the problem and the purpose significant? Provide a rationale.

4. Does the purpose identify the variables, population, and setting for this study?
   a. Identify the variables:

   b. Identify the population:

   c. Identify the setting:

5. Are the problem and purpose feasible for the researchers to study? Provide a rationale.

Lewis, *et al.* Study

♦ **Directions:** Review the Lewis *et al.* (1997) article in Appendix B and answer the following questions.

1. State the problem addressed in this study.

2. State the purpose of this study.

3. Are the problem and the purpose significant? Provide a rationale.

4. Does the purpose identify the variables, population, and setting for this study?
   a. Identify the variables:

   b. Identify the population:

   c. Identify the setting:

5. Are the problem and purpose feasible for the researchers to study? Provide a rationale.

Bruce & Grove Study

♦ **Directions:** Review the Bruce & Grove (1994) article in Appendix B and answer the following questions.

1. State the problem addressed in this study.

2. State the purpose of this study.

3. Are the problem and the purpose significant? Provide a rationale.

4. Does the purpose identify the variables, population, and setting for this study?
    a. Identify the variables:

    b. Identify the population:

    c. Identify the setting:

5. Are the problem and purpose feasible for the researchers to study? Provide a rationale.

⌘ MAKING CONNECTIONS

Objectives, Questions, and Hypotheses

♦ **Directions:** Identify each of the ten example hypotheses using the terms listed below. Four terms are needed to identify each hypothesis. The correct answer for hypothesis #1 is provided as an example.

a. associative hypothesis
b. causal hypothesis
c. complex hypothesis
d. directional hypothesis

e. nondirectional hypothesis
f. null hypothesis
g. research hypothesis
h. simple hypothesis

b, c, d, g   1. Relaxation therapy is more effective than standard care in decreasing pain perception and use of pain medications in adults with chronic arthritic pain.

_____ 2. Age, family support, and health status are related to the self-care abilities of nursing home residents.

_____ 3. Heparinized saline is no more effective than normal saline in maintaining the patency and comfort of a heparin lock.

_____ 4. Poor health status is related to decreasing self-care abilities in institutionalized elderly patients.

_____ 5. Low-back massage is more effective in decreasing perception of low-back pain than no massage in patients with chronic low-back pain.

_____ 6. Healthy adults involved in a diet and exercise program have lower low-density lipoprotein (LDL), higher high-density lipoprotein (HDL), and lower cardiovascular risk levels than adults not involved in the program.

_____ 7. Time on the operating table, diastolic blood pressure, age, and preoperative albumin levels are related to development of pressure ulcers in hospitalized elderly patients.

_____ 8. There are no differences in complications or incidence of phlebitis in heparin locks changed every 72 hours and those locks left in place up to 168 hours.

_____ 9. Nurses' perceived work stress, internal locus of control, and social support are related to their psychological symptoms.

_____ 10. Cancer patients with chronic pain who listen to music with positive suggestion of pain reduction have less pain than those who do not listen to music.

11. State hypothesis #5 as a null hypothesis.

12. State hypothesis #2 as a directional hypothesis.

13. State hypothesis #9 as a null hypothesis.

⌘ EXERCISES IN CRITIQUE

Berg, *et al.* Study

♦ **Directions:** Review the Berg, *et al.* (1997) article in Appendix B and answer the following questions.

1. Are objectives, questions, or hypotheses stated in this study? _____

    Identify these:

2. Are these appropriate and clearly stated? Provide a rationale.

Lewis, *et al.* Study

♦ **Directions:** Review the Lewis, *et al.* (1997) article in Appendix B and answer the following questions.

1. Are objectives, questions, or hypotheses stated in this study? _____

   Identify these:

2. Are these appropriate and clearly stated? Provide a rationale.

Bruce & Grove Study

♦ **Directions:** Review the Bruce and Grove (1994) article in Appendix B and answer the following questions.

1. Are objectives, questions, or hypotheses stated in this study? _____

   Identify these:

2. Are these appropriate and clearly stated? Provide a rationale.

⌘ MAKING CONNECTIONS

Understanding Study Variables

◆ **Directions:** Match each type of variable with the example variables provided below.

     a. demographic variable
     b. dependent variable
     c. independent variable

____ 1. age

____ 2. perception of pain

____ 3. exercise program

____ 4. gender

____ 5. length of hospital stay

____ 6. incidence of phlebitis

____ 7. relaxation therapy

____ 8. low-back massage

____ 9. educational level

____ 10. postoperative pain

____ 11. ethnic background

____ 12. marital status

⌘ EXERCISES IN CRITIQUE

Berg *et al.* Study

◆ **Directions:** Read the Berg, *et al.* (1997) article and answer the following questions.

1. List the major variables in this study and identify the type of variable (independent, dependent, or research).

    Type of Variable   *Variable*

2. Identify the conceptual and operational definitions for the self-management program and compliance with inhaled medications variables.

3. Are these definitions clear? Provide a rationale.

Lewis, *et al.* Study

♦ **Directions:** Read the Lewis, *et al.* (1997) article and answer the following questions.

1. List the major variables in this article and identify the type of variable (independent, dependent, or research).

    Type of Variable   *Variable*

2. Identify the conceptual and operational definitions for the variable body position (right or left lateral).

3. Is this definition clear? Provide a rationale.

Bruce & Grove Study

♦ **Directions:** Read the Bruce & Grove (1994) article and answer the following questions.

1. List the major variables in this study and identify the type of variable (independent, dependent, or research).

   Type of Variable   *Variable*

2. Identify the conceptual and operational definitions for the CARE program variable.

3. Are these definitions clear? Provide a rationale.

CHAPTER 4
REVIEW OF LITERATURE

⌘ INTRODUCTION

Read Chapter 4 and then complete the following exercises. These exercises will assist you in reading and critiquing research reports and summarizing the findings for use in practice. The answers to these exercises are in Appendix A under Chapter 4.

⌘ RELEVANT TERMS

♦ **Directions:** Match each term below with its correct definition.

a. academic library
b. approximate replication
c. computer search
d. concurrent replication
e. databases
f. dissertation
g. empirical literature
h. exact replication
i. integrative review of research

j. interlibrary loan department
k. primary source
l. review of literature
m. secondary source
n. special library
o. systematic extension replication
p. theoretical literature
q. thesis
r. World Wide Web (WWW)

Definitions

_____ 1. Source whose author summarizes or quotes content from a primary source.
_____ 2. Department that locates books and articles in other libraries and provides the sources within a designated time.
_____ 3. Constructive replication performed under distinctly new conditions, in which the researchers conducting the replication do not follow the design or methods of the original research; rather, the second investigative team begins with a similar problem statement but formulates new means to verify the first investigator's findings.

___ 4. Literature that includes concept analyses, maps, theories, and conceptual frameworks that support a selected research problem and purpose.

___ 5. Structured compilation of information that can be scanned, retrieved, and analyzed by computer and can be used for decisions, reports, and research.

___ 6. Source whose author originated or is responsible for generating the ideas published.

___ 7. Library that contains a collection of materials on a specific topic or specialty area, such as a library associated with a hospital.

___ 8. Internal replication that involves the collection of data for the original study and its replication simultaneously to provide a check of the reliability of the original study findings.

___ 9. Review conducted to identify, analyze, and synthesize the results from independent studies to determine the current knowledge in a particular area.

___ 10. Function conducted to scan the citations in different databases and identify sources relevant to a selected topic.

___ 11. Review of theoretical and empirical sources to generate a picture of what is known and not known about a problem that provides a basis of the study conducted.

___ 12. A research project completed by a student as part of the requirements for a master's degree.

___ 13. An information service for access to the Internet resources by content rather than file names.

___ 14. Precise duplication of the initial researcher's study to confirm the original findings.

___ 15. Relevant studies published in journals and books; also includes unpublished studies such as master's theses and doctoral dissertations.

___ 16. Library located within an institution of higher learning that contains numerous journals and books.

___ 17. Operational replication that involves repeating the original study under similar conditions, following the methods as closely as possible.

___ 18. An extensive, usually original research project that is completed by a doctoral student as part of the requirements for a doctoral degree.

⌘ KEY IDEAS

♦ **Directions:** Fill in the blanks with the appropriate word(s).

1. Predominately two types of sources are reviewed and cited in a literature review; these

   are _____ and _____ sources.

2. The purpose for conducting a literature review in phenomenological research is to

   _____

   _____ .

3. The review of literature is conducted to provide a background for the conduct of a study in _____ and _____.

4. The literature is reviewed to develop research questions and is a source of data in

   _____ .

5. Williams' (1972) study, conducted to examine factors that contribute to skin breakdown, is considered a _____ study in the area of pressure ulcer prevention.

6. Studies need to be _____ to determine if the findings are consistent from one study to another.

7. Researchers are conducting an _____ replication of a study if they are repeating the study using different subjects and measuring the variables with improved methods of measurement.

8. Is this textbook, *Understanding Nursing Research,* an example of a primary or secondary source? _____

9. Identify, in correct order, the four steps for reviewing the literature.

   a. _____

   b. _____

   c. _____

   d. _____

10. Two important libraries for locating research publications in journals and books are

    _____ and _____.

11. Manual search of the literature involves examining:

    a. _____

    b. _____

    c. _____

    d. _____

12. The most important index for locating nursing sources is the

    _____ .

13. The _____ is a worldwide network that connects computers together.

14. Identify two of the databases commonly used by nurses to locate relevant sources.

    a. _____

    b. _____

15. The _____ is a good source for integrative reviews of research relevant to nursing practice.

16. Reviewing the literature requires a _____ of research sources to determine what is known and not known about a clinical problem.

17. The review of literature for use of study findings in practice usually includes the following sections: _____, _____ _____, and _____.

18. Given the research problem that "Although core rewarming is initiated prior to removal from the cardiopulmonary bypass machine (CPB), severe peripheral hypothermia and vasoconstriction often persist into the postoperative period" (Giuffre, M., Heidenreich, T., & Pruitt, L. (1994). Rewarming cardiac surgery patients: Radiant heat versus forced warm air. *Nursing Research, 43*(3), p. 174). What key terms would you use to direct your review of literature for this problem?

19. Given the research problem that "Urinary incontinence is a common problem among nursing home (NH) residents and can be successfully treated with prompted voiding during daytime hours . . . Nighttime incontinence care should be individualized to minimize sleep disruption while considering moisture exposure that could affect skin health. Although descriptive studies have been published, there are no published intervention studies describing attempts to improve nighttime environmental factors in NHs" (p. 197). (Schnelle, J.F., Cruise, P.A., Alessi, C.A., Al-Samarrai, N., & Ouslander, J.G.

(1998). Individualizing nighttime incontinence care in nursing home residents. *Nursing Research, 47*(4), 197–204). What key terms would you use to direct your review of literature for this problem?

20. List the three steps for locating research sources.

a. _____

b. _____

c. _____

⌘ MAKING CONNECTIONS

Theoretical and Empirical Sources

♦ **Directions:** Theoretical and empirical literature are included in the literature review of a published study. Read the sources below and identify the sources that are theoretical with a **T** and the sources that are empirical with an **E.**

_____ 1. Lazarus and Folkman's Theory of Coping

_____ 2. abstracts from a research conference

_____ 3. theses

_____ 4. Watson's philosophy of human caring

_____ 5. Orem, D.E. (1991). *Nursing: Concepts of practice* (4th ed.) St. Louis: Mosby.

_____ 6. Giuffre, M., Heidenreich, T., & Pruitt, L. (1994). Rewarming cardiac surgery patients: Radiant heat versus warm air. *Nursing Research, 43*(3), 174–178.

_____ 7. Lowry, L.W., & Beikirch, P. (1998). Effects of comprehensive care on pregnancy outcomes. *Applied Nursing Research, 11*(2), 55–61.

_____ 8. dissertations

_____ 9. von Bertalanffy, L. (1968). *General systems theory.* New York: Braziller.

_____ 10. Lewin's Change Theory

_____ 11. Burns, N., Carney, K., & Slinkman, C. (1998). Development of the rural-urban demand indicator. *Research in Nursing & Health, 21*(5), 453–466.

Primary and Secondary Sources

♦ **Directions:** A literature review includes mainly primary sources. Label the primary sources below with a **P** and the secondary sources with an **S.**

_____ 1. integrated review of research

_____ 2. dissertations

_____ 3. theses

_____ 4. textbooks

_____ 5. summary of theoretical and empirical sources

_____ 6. study published in *Applied Nursing Research*

_____ 7. landmark study of pressure ulcers

_____ 8. published review of literature article

_____ 9. exact replication of a study

_____ 10. historical research article in *Image: Journal of Nursing Scholarship*

⌘ EXERCISES IN CRITIQUE

♦ **Directions:** Review the three articles in Appendix B and use these articles to answer the following questions.

1. The most common format for citing a reference is the American Psychological Association (APA) (1994) format. Knowing the different parts of a reference citation will assist you in locating and recording sources for a formal paper. The following source is presented in APA format.

   Bruce, S.L., & Grove, S.K. (1994). The effect of a coronary artery risk evaluation program on serum lipid values and cardiovascular risk levels. *Applied Nursing Research,* 7(2), 67–74.

   a. In this reference, *Applied Nursing Research* is the _____.

   b. In this reference, the 1994 is _____.

   c. In this reference, the 7 is the _____.

   d. In this reference, the 67–74 is the _____.

   e. In this reference, the 2 is the _____.

   f. Who are the authors of this article? _____ and _____

   g. What is the title of the article? _____
   _____

2. Write the reference for the Berg, Dunbar-Jacob, & Sereika (1997) article using APA format.

_____

_____

_____

3. If the reference citations below are not complete, indicate what is missing. Incomplete references in published studies are a problem for people trying to locate sources from the reference list of the article.

   a. Christman, S.K., Fish, A.F., Frid, D.J., Smith, B.A., & Bryant, C.X. (1998). *Applied Nursing Research, 7*(2).
   What is missing?

   b. Anderson, M.A., & Helms, L.B. (1998). Extended care referral after hospital discharge. *Research in Nursing & Health,* (5).
   What is missing?

   c. Schlenk, E.A., & Boehm, S. Behaviors in type II diabetes during contingency contracting. *Applied Nursing Research,* 77–83.
   What is missing?

4. What are the titles for the literature review section in the three articles in Appendix B?
   a. Berg, *et al.* (1997)

   _____

   b. Lewis, *et al.* (1997)

   _____

   c. Bruce & Grove (1994)

   _____

5. Are relevant studies identified and described in the Berg, *et al.* (1997) literature review? Give two examples of studies that are cited in the literature review of the article.

6. Are relevant theories identified and described in the Berg, *et al.* (1997) study? Identify one theoretical source that is cited in the study's literature review.

7. In the references for the Berg, *et al.* (1997) study, is the source by Coutts, Gibson, and

   Paton (1990) a primary or secondary source? _____

8. Which of the sources in the References section of the Berg, *et al.* (1997) study is an integrated review of the literature?

9. Are the references in the Berg, *et al.* (1997) study current? Provide a rationale.

10. Does the literature review in the Berg, *et al.* (1997) study present the current knowledge base for the research problem? Provide a rationale.

11. Are relevant studies identified and described in the Lewis, *et al.* (1997) study? Give two examples of studies that are cited in the literature review of the article.

12. Are relevant theories identified and described in the Lewis, *et al.* (1997) study? Identify one theoretical source that is cited in the study's literature review.

13. In the Lewis, *et al.,* (1997) study references, is the source by Luckmann & Sorensen (1993) a primary or secondary source? _____ Is the source by Shinners & Pease (1993) a primary or secondary source? _____

14. Are the references in the Lewis, *et al.* (1997) study current? Provide a rationale.

15. Does the literature review in the Lewis, *et al.* (1997) study provide a current knowledge base for the research problem examined in this study? Provide a rationale.

16. Are relevant studies identified and described in the Bruce & Grove (1994) study? Give two examples of studies that are cited in the literature review of the article.

17. Are relevant theories identified and described in the Bruce & Grove (1994) study? Identify one theoretical source that is cited in the study's literature review.

18. In Bruce & Grove's references, is the source by Glanz (1988) a primary or secondary source? _____ Is the source by Blair, Bryant, & Bocuzzi (1988) a primary or secondary source? _____

19. Are the references in the Bruce & Grove (1994) study current? Provide a rationale.

20. Does the literature review of Bruce & Grove's (1994) study provide a current knowledge base for the research problem examined in this study? Provide a rationale.

⌘ GOING BEYOND

♦ **Directions:** Identify a problem in clinical practice and conduct a summary of the research literature on this topic.

1. Search the literature for relevant research sources. Has an integrative review been done on this topic? Review Appendix 3a of your textbook for a list of integrated reviews of nursing research.
2. Locate relevant studies in your university library.
3. Read each study and identify the steps of the research process.
4. Outline key information from each study, including the study purpose, framework, sample size, design, results, and findings.
5. Critique the quality of each study.
6. Write a description of each research report and critique the quality of the report.
7. Write a summary paragraph that indicates what is known and not known about the clinical problem you selected.
8. Ask your instructor to evaluate your review of the research literature.

CHAPTER 5
UNDERSTANDING THEORY AND
RESEARCH FRAMEWORKS

⌘ INTRODUCTION

Read Chapter 5 and then complete the following exercises. These exercises will assist you in learning relevant terms and identifying and critiquing frameworks in published studies. The answers to these exercises are in Appendix A under Chapter 5.

⌘ RELEVANT TERMS

♦ **Directions:** Define the following terms in your own words without looking at your textbook. Then check your definitions with those in the glossary of your textbook. Using this strategy, you can identify elements of the terms that are not yet clear in your mind. Reread the appropriate sections of the chapter to clarify your understanding of each term.

1. abstract _____

   _____

2. concept _____

   _____

3. conceptual definition _____

   _____

4. concrete _____

   _____

5. conceptual model _____

   _____

6. construct _____

_____

7. existence statement _____

_____

8. hypotheses _____

_____

9. relational statement _____

_____

10. proposition _____

_____

11. theory _____

_____

12. variable _____

_____

⌘ KEY IDEAS

♦ **Directions:** Fill in the blanks with the appropriate word(s) or numbers.

1. We use theories to _____ .

2. Testing a theory involves _____

_____ .

3. _____ are not generally considered testable.

4. Research is based on _____ .

5. A framework that has been used rather shallowly to provide an overall orientation for a study but does not guide the study is referred to as _____ .

6. Research findings are interpreted in terms of _____ .

7. In a framework, all _____ should be defined.

8. Concepts in conceptual models are referred to as _____ .

9. A _____ is more specific than a concept and is defined so that it is measurable.

10. The _____ of a theory are tested through research.

11. Statements at the lowest level of abstraction are referred to as

_____ .

12. The purpose of a conceptual map is to _____

_____ .

13. A conceptual map includes _____

_____ .

14. An organized program of research designed to build a body of knowledge related to a particular conceptual model is referred to as a _____ .

⌘ MAKING CONNECTIONS

♦ **Directions:** Match the following ideas.

_____ 1. theory   a. broadly explains phenomena of interest
_____ 2. concept   b. the basic element of a theory
_____ 3. conceptual model   c. expresses a claim important to a theory
_____ 4. variable   d. graphically shows interrelations among concepts
_____ 5. statement   e. integrated set of defined concepts and statements
_____ 6. conceptual map   f. statement expressed at low level of abstraction
_____ 7. framework   g. provides general meanings of terms
_____ 8. construct   h. defines a term so that it is measurable
_____ 9. hypothesis   i. presents portions of a theory to be tested in a study

⌘ PUZZLES

Word Scramble

♦ **Directions:** Unscramble the words in the following sentence to determine its meaning.

Amyn tusidse rea duirqere to diavelat lal of eht tesnamtets ni a yrehto.

Secret Message

Aqw pggf vq fgvgtokpg nkpmu coqpi vjg eqpegrvwcn fghkpkvkqpu, vjg xctkcdngu kp vjg

uvwfa, cpf vjg tgncvgf ogcuwtgogpv ogvjqfu.

Crossword Puzzle

♦ **Directions:** Complete the crossword puzzle. Note that if the answer is more than one word, there are no blank spaces left between words.

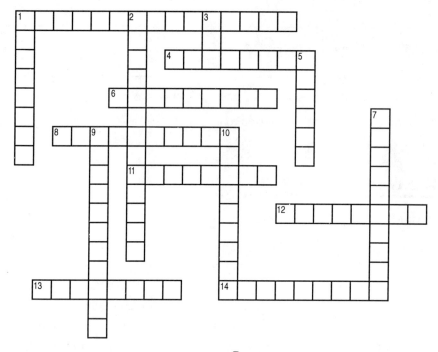

Across

1. not considered testable through research
4. framework with ideas not fully developed
6. portion of a theory to be tested in a study
8. specific statement expressed at lowest level of abstraction
11. focus of Orem's model
12. expression of an idea apart from any specific instance
13. term in which numerical values vary from one instance to another
14. an organized program of research designed to build a body of knowledge related to a particular conceptual model

Down

1. ideas concerned with realities or actual instances
2. process of determining the truth of a relational statement
3. developed to explain which concepts contribute to or partially cause an outcome
5. used to describe, explain, predict, and/or control a phenomenon
7. focus of Roy's model
9. statement found in theories
10. clarifies the type of relationship that exists between or among concepts

⌘ EXERCISES IN CRITIQUE

♦ **Directions:** Examine the framework of Lewis, Nichols, Mackey, Fadol, Sloane, Villagomez, & Liehr's study in Appendix B.

1. List the concepts in the study.

2. State the definition of each concept as defined by the author(s). Are the definitions clear and adequate? If not, identify the inadequacies.

3. Complete the following table by listing each concept, its related variable(s), and its measurement method.

CONCEPT	VARIABLE	MEASUREMENT

4. Compare the measurement method for each variable with its associated concept and conceptual definition. Is each measurement method consistent with its associated concept and conceptual definition? If not, what is/are the inconsistencies?

5. List the statements expressed within the publication. Underline the concepts included in each statement. Are all of the study concepts included within a statement? Provide a map of each statement.

6. State the proposition(s) being tested in the study and the related hypothesis or research question.

7. Are the statements tested by the study design? How?

8. Is the framework expressed as a conceptual map? Are all of the concepts in the study included in the map? Are all of the statements you identified included in the map? If there is no map, develop one and draw it here.

9. Does the author provide statements for each linkage between concepts shown on the map? Does the author provide references from the literature to support the linkages? List the references for each linkage.

10. Develop a short summary paragraph describing the strengths and weaknesses of the framework.

⌘ GOING BEYOND

1. Berg's study has an implicit framework. Using the above questions, extract the framework.
2. The framework for Bruce & Grove's study was removed by the editors prior to publication. Try to construct a framework for their study from the introduction and literature review.

CHAPTER 6
EXAMINING ETHICS IN
NURSING RESEARCH

⌘ INTRODUCTION

Read Chapter 6 and then complete the following exercises. These exercises will assist you in understanding the ethical aspects of studies. The answers to these exercises are in Appendix A under Chapter 6.

⌘ RELEVANT TERMS

♦ **Directions:** Match each term with its correct definition.

a. anonymity	g. informed consent
b. benefit-risk ratio	h. institutional review
c. confidentiality	i. nontherapeutic research
d. discomfort and harm	j. Privacy Act
e. ethical principles	k. scientific misconduct
f. human rights	l. therapeutic research

Definitions

_____ 1. Claims and demands that have been justified in the eyes of an individual or by the consensus of a group of individuals and are protected in research.

_____ 2. Condition in which a subject's identity cannot be linked, even by the researcher, with his or her individual responses.

_____ 3. Agreement by a prospective subject to participate voluntarily in a study after he or she has assimilated essential information about the study.

_____ 4. Research conducted to generate knowledge for a discipline; the results might benefit future patients but will probably not benefit the research subjects.

_____ 5. Process of examining studies for ethical concerns by a committee of peers.

_____ 6. Phrase used to describe the degree of risk for a subject participating in a study. The levels of risk include: no anticipated effects, temporary discomfort, unusual levels of temporary discomfort, risk of permanent damage, and certainty of permanent damage.

_____ 7. Freedom of an individual to determine the time, extent, and general circumstances under which private information will be shared with or withheld from others.

_____ 8. Ratio considered by researchers and reviewers of research as they weigh potential benefits and risks in a study to promote the conduct of ethical research.

_____ 9. Research that provides a patient with an opportunity to receive an experimental treatment that might have beneficial results.

_____ 10. Principles of respect for persons, beneficence, and justice that are relevant to the conduct of research.

_____ 11. Management of private data in research in such a way that subjects' identities are not linked with their responses.

_____ 12. Practices such as fabrication, falsification, or forging of data; dishonest manipulation of the study design or methods; and plagiarism.

⌘ KEY IDEAS

♦ **Directions:** Fill in the blanks with the correct responses.

1. The elements of informed consent include:

   a. _____

   b. _____

   c. _____

   d. _____

2. Identify six types of information that must be included in the consent form.

   a. _____

   b. _____

   c. _____

   d. _____

   e. _____

   f. _____

3. _____ consent means that the prospective subject has decided to take part in a study of his or her own volition without coercion or any undue influence.

4. Subjects with diminished autonomy, *e.g.,* children and people with mental illnesses, are vulnerable and _____ to consent to participate in research.

5. Before a study is conducted, it must be reviewed by a committee of peers, which is called an _____.

6. The three levels of institutional review of research are:

   a. _____

   b. _____

   c. _____

7. How do you assess the benefit-risk ratio of a published study?

8. What type of institutional review would a study probably require if it involved the review of patients' records to identify their fasting blood sugar value prior to surgery?

   _____

9. A study that involved examining the effects of a new drug on patients' serum lipid values would probably require what type of institutional review? _____

10. Identify three different types of scientific misconduct.

   a. _____

   b. _____

   c. _____

11. The names of the two federal agencies that were organized for reporting and
    investigating scientific misconduct are: _____

    and _____ .

12. Is scientific misconduct present in nursing? _____

13. Are animals used in research conducted by nurses? _____

14. This agency was developed to ensure the humane treatment of animals in research:

    _____

15. Should animals be used as research subjects? Provide a rationale for your response.

⌘ MAKING CONNECTIONS

Historical Events, Ethical Codes, and Regulation

♦ **Directions:** Match the unethical studies listed below with the correct descriptions.

    a. Jewish Chronic Disease Hospital study
    b. Nazi medical experiments
    c. Tuskegee syphilis study
    d. Willowbrook study

_____ 1. Subjects were exposed to freezing temperatures, high altitudes, poisons, untested
      drugs, and experimental operations.
_____ 2. Study was conducted to determine the natural course of syphilis in the adult, black
      male.
_____ 3. Subjects were deliberately infected with the hepatitis virus in this study.
_____ 4. Subjects were frequently killed or sustained permanent physical, mental, or social
      damage during these studies.
_____ 5. Subjects did not receive penicillin when it was identified as an effective treatment
      for their disease.
_____ 6. The purpose of this study was to determine the patients' rejection responses to live
      cancer cells.
_____ 7. The subjects in this study were institutionalized, mentally retarded children.
_____ 8. These experiments resulted in the development of the Nuremberg Code.
_____ 9. The subjects were injected with live cancer cells without their knowledge.
_____ 10. This study continued until 1972 when an account of the study appeared in the
      Washington Star and public outrage demanded that the study be stopped.

⌘ PUZZLES

Crossword

♦ **Directions:** Complete the crossword puzzle. Note that if the answer is more than one word, there are no blank spaces left between words.

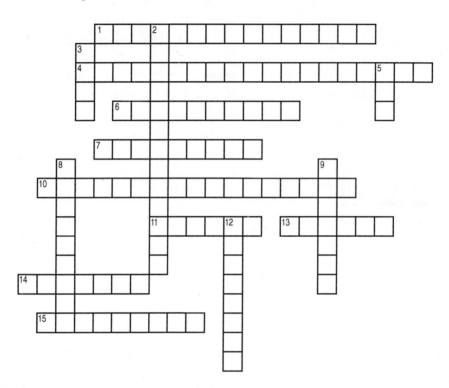

Across
1. keeping data private
4. agency evaluation of a study to protect potential subjects
6. subjects who can legally choose to participate or not in a study are ____
7. code developed after World War II
10. controlling your own fate
11. focuses on human rights of research
13. child's agreement to be in a study
14. ____ Act of 1974
15. identity of subjects unknown

Down
2. Subjects should receive ____ ____ during a study.
3. opposite of benefit that must be examined to determine if a study is ethical
5. Institutional Review Board
8. misinforming subjects
9. subject's permission to be in a study
12. incompetent to give consent

⌘ EXERCISES IN CRITIQUE

♦ **Directions:** Review the research articles in Appendix B to answer the following questions.

1. Is the Berg, Dunbar-Jacob, & Sereika (1997) study ethical? Identify the information in the study that indicates that the subjects' rights were protected and institutional review was obtained.

2. Is the Lewis, Nichols, Mackey, Fadol, Sloane, Villagomez, & Liehr (1997) study ethical? Identify the information in the study that indicates that the subjects' rights were protected and institutional review was obtained.

3. Is the Bruce & Grove (1994) study ethical? Identify the information in the study that indicates that the subjects' rights were protected and institutional review was obtained.

CHAPTER 7
CLARIFYING RESEARCH DESIGNS

⌘ INTRODUCTION

Read Chapter 7 and then complete the following exercises. These exercises will assist you in learning relevant terms and identifying and critiquing designs in published studies. The answers to these exercises are in Appendix A under Chapter 7.

⌘ RELEVANT TERMS

♦ **Directions:** Define the following terms in your own words without looking at your textbook. Then check your definitions with those in the glossary of your textbook. Using this strategy, you can identify elements of the terms that are not yet clear in your mind. Reread the appropriate sections of the chapter to clarify your understanding of each term.

1. bias _____

   _____

2. causality _____

   _____

3. control _____

   _____

4. design validity _____

   _____

5. external validity _____

   _____

6. heterogeneity _____

   _____

7. homogeneity _____

   _____

8. internal validity _____

   _____

9. manipulation _____

   _____

10. multicausality _____

    _____

11. probability _____

    _____

⌘ KEY IDEAS

♦ **Directions:** Fill in the blanks with the appropriate word(s) or numbers.

1. According to causality theory, things have causes and causes lead to

   _____.

2. From the perspective of probability, a _____ may not

   produce a specific _____ each time that particular

   _____ occurs.

3. Designs are developed to reduce the possibilities and effects of

   _____.

4. The purpose of research designs is to maximize _____

   factors in the study situation.

5. The most commonly used manipulation in a study is the

   _____.

6. Critical analysis of research involves being able to think through _____

_____ that have occurred and make judgments

about how seriously these affect the integrity of the findings.

7. Quasi-experimental and experimental studies are designed to examine

_____.

8. In most studies, _____ are the basis of obtaining valid

answers.

9. Designs were developed to reduce threats to the validity of the

_____.

⌘ MAKING CONNECTIONS

Matching Definitions

♦ **Directions:** Match the following terms with their correct definitions.

_____ 1. design validity
_____ 2. multicausality
_____ 3. descriptive design
_____ 4. bias
_____ 5. control
_____ 6. internal validity
_____ 7. probability
_____ 8. external validity
_____ 9. correlational design

a. to deviate from the true or expected

b. the extent to which study findings can be generalized beyond the sample used in the study

c. extent to which the effects detected in the study are a true reflection of reality

d. addresses relative causality

e. to examine relationships between or among two or more variables in a single group

f. the power to direct or manipulate factors to achieve a desired outcome

g. the study provides a convincing test of the framework propositions

h. the recognition that a number of interrelating variables can be involved in causing a particular effect

i. to gain more information about characteristics in a particular field of study

Matching Designs

♦ **Directions:** Match each design type with the corresponding study description.

a. typical descriptive study design
b. comparative descriptive design
c. longitudinal design
d. trend design
e. case study design

f. descriptive correlational design
g. predictive correlational design
h. model testing design
i. quasi-experimental design
j. experimental design

_____ 1. The purpose of this study was to describe the physical status, emotional state (depression and motivation), and functional performance of residents in a long-term care facility and to explore the impact of motivation (intrinsic and extrinsic factors), demographic variables, length of time institutionalized, physical status, depression, and fear of falling on functional performance of older adults in a long-term care setting (Resnick, 1998, p. 231).

_____ 2. Annual self-assessments of MS [multiple sclerosis]-related symptoms and level of ADL [activities of daily living] functioning were used to examine the chronic illness trajectory over a 10-year period (Gulick, 1998, p. 138).

_____ 3. The purpose of the study was to describe the relationships among perceived social support, uncertainty, and psychological distress in adolescents recently diagnosed with cancer (Neville, 1998, p. 38).

_____ 4. The purpose of this study is to examine patient characteristics that predict referral to outpatient CR [cardiac rehabilitation] following hospitalization for MI [myocardial infarction] or CABG [coronary artery bypass surgery] (Burns, Camaione, Froman, & Clark, 1998, p. 148).

_____ 5. The purpose of this study was to describe and compare differences in demographics, prenatal care use, and pregnancy, labor, postpartum, and neonatal complications for 129 pregnant Mexican-American adolescents who were either born in the United States or born in Mexico (Koshar, Lee, Goss, Heilemann, & Stinson, 1998).

_____ 6. The purpose of the study was to examine the effects of ovarian hormone cessation, hormone supplementation, and dietary fiber composition on body weight, appetite, and intestinal transit. In Part 1, effects of ovarian hormone status on body weight and baseline and stimulated intestinal transit were measured in chow-fed rats. Sprague-Dawley rats were ovariectomized (OVX), then injected daily (22 days) with estrogen (E), progesterone (P), the combination (E+P), or placebo. Controls were sham operated and placebo injected (Bond Heitkemper, & Jarrett, 1994, p. 18).

_____ 7. The purpose of this study was to describe and analyze events occurring to a single patient who experienced hypokalemic periodic paralysis (Anderson, 1998).

_____ 8. The purpose of this study was to compare the safety of automatic blood pressure cuffs versus manual cuffs when used on patients receiving thrombolytic therapy. This prospective, randomized trial compared manual and automatic devices for measuring blood pressure. A convenience sample was used to study patients in 8 hospitals throughout the United States (Saul, Smith, & Mook, 1998, p. 193).

_____ 9. The purpose of this study was to develop and examine the predictive ability of a model of exercise among older adults (Conn, 1998, p. 180).

_____ 10. This paper shows the infant mortality rates (IMR) for all of Queensland, and at Cherbourg from 1910 to 1990 and the weights of four cohorts of children at Cherbourg over 40 years (Alsop-Shields, 1998).

Mapping the Design

♦ **Directions:** Map the design for the following quasi-experimental studies.

1. The purpose of the study was to investigate the effects of a transmural home care intervention program for terminal cancer patients on the direct caregivers' (the patient's principal informal caregivers') quality of life, compared with standard care programs. The intervention program intended to optimize the cooperation and coordination between the intramural and extramural health care organizations (transmural care). Direct caregivers of terminal cancer patients (estimated prognosis less than 6 months) could be included in this quasi-experimental study. The direct caregivers' quality of life was measured in a multidimensional way 1 week before (T1), 1 week after (T2), and 4 weeks after (T3) the patient's discharge from the hospital (discharge being the starting point of the intervention), then again at 3 months after the patient's death (T4) (Smeenk, de Witte, van Haastragt, Schipper, Beizemans, & Crebolder, 1998, p. 129) . . . Direct caregivers of patients fulfilling the inclusion criteria and living in Eindhoven, The Netherlands, were allocated to the intervention group and those living in the urban surroundings of Eindhoven were allocated to the control group. After the patients' discharge from the hospital (*i.e.,* the start of the intervention), patients and their direct caregivers in both groups received the standard care available in The Netherlands (Schrijvers, 1997). In addition to this care, patients and their direct caregivers allocated to the intervention group were offered the intervention program (p. 130).

2. Objectives: To test a structured communications program for family members to determine whether the program would increase family members' satisfaction with care, meet their needs for information better, and decrease disruption for the ICU nursing staff caused by incoming telephone calls from patients' family members (p. 24) . . . The groups consisted of family members of patients in a medical ICU. Only one medical ICU was used, so that the setting and personnel would not differ between the two groups. The experimental group received the structured communication program, and the control group received usual care. Pretest data were collected approximately 24 hours after the patient was admitted to the medical ICU. Posttest data were collected on the day of discharge from the unit or 2 weeks after admission to the unit for those patients who had not been discharged yet. The same instruments were administered before and after the intervention (pretest and posttest) to both groups. To prevent contamination between groups, we collected data for the control group first. After the control-group phase was finished, the nature of the intervention was explained to the ICU nurses and the intervention phase was started (Medland, Ferrans, & the College of Nursing, University of Illinois at Chicago, 1998, p. 25).

3. A method of multidisciplinary care delivery was designed that included an outcomes manager, a care pathway for patients receiving mechanical ventilation, and weaning protocols. Data collection consisted of three parts: a retrospective review of 124 patients who required prolonged ventilation during a 1-year period before implementation of the care model, a 6-month prospective study in which 91 patients were alternately assigned by month to an outcomes-managed approach or a non-outcomes-managed approach, and a 6-month prospective study of 90 patients in which an outcomes-managed approach without alternate-month assignment was used (Burns, Marshall, Ryan, Wilmoth, Carpenter, Alio, Wood, & Truwitt, 1998, p. 45).

⌘ PUZZLES

Word Scramble

♦ **Directions:** Unscramble the words in the following sentences to determine their meaning.

Sjut sa hte libunetpr rof a usheo tmus eb vidnuizliddaie to eth fseccipi esuho giben itlub, os tsum eht snedig eb daem piseccif ot a yudst.

Secret Message

Ymj uzwutxj tk f ijxnls nx yt xjy zu f xnyzfynts ymfy rfcnrnejx ymj utxxngnqnynjx tk tgyfnsnsl fhhzwfyj fsxajwx yt tgojhynajx, vzjxynts, tw mdutymjxjx.

Crossword Puzzle

♦ **Directions:** Complete the crossword puzzle. Note that if the answer is more than one word, there are no blank spaces left between the words.

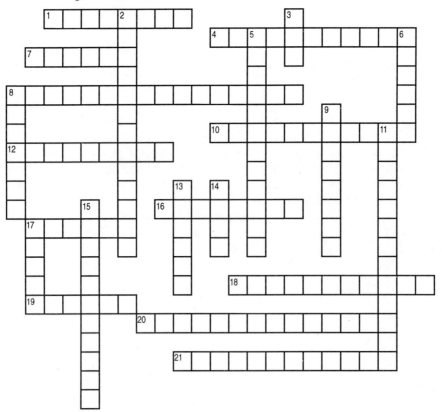

Across

1. selection of a control group subject who has similar characteristics to an experimental group subject
4. a good design reduces threats to the validity of these
7. a cause leads to this
8. administration of multiple treatments in random order
10. the purpose of sampling criteria is to establish this among subjects
12. independent variable
16. an examination of whether the study provides a convincing test of the framework propositions
17. a danger to the integrity of the findings
18. relative, rather than absolute, causality
19. blueprint for conducting a study
20. design strategy used to ensure even distribution of important variables throughout the sample
21. designs that provide greatest control in examining effects

Down

2. a design strategy in which subjects with a wide variety of characteristics are obtained
3. a visual depiction of the design
5. to move around or control movement
6. group of subjects selected for a study
8. imposing of rules in a design
9. controls the number of subjects at various levels of an extraneous variable in a sample
11. designs used to examine relationships between or among two or more variables in single group
13. strategy used to increase probability of equivalence of sample with population
14. deviation of findings from the true
15. design used to provide a picture of situations as they naturally happen
17. Design used to examine changes in the general population

⌘ EXERCISES IN CRITIQUE

♦ **Directions:** Review the research articles in Appendix B and answer the following questions.

1. Identify the design used in:

    a. Berg, Dunbar-Jacob, & Sereika's study _____

    b. Lewis & colleagues' study _____

    c. Bruce & Grove's study _____

2. Identify three sources of potential bias in the study design of:

    a. Berg, Dunbar-Jacob, & Sereika's study _____

    _____

    _____

    b. Lewis & colleagues' study _____

_____

_____

    c. Bruce & Grove's study _____

_____

_____

3. List three methods of control used in the design of:

    a. Berg, Dunbar-Jacob, & Sereika's study _____

_____

_____

    b. Lewis & colleagues' study _____

_____

_____

    c. Bruce & Grove's study _____

_____

_____

4. What comparisons could be made given the design used in:

    a. Berg, Dunbar-Jacob, & Sereika's study

    b. Lewis & colleagues' study

    c. Bruce & Grove's study

5. To what populations can the findings be generalized from:

   a. Berg, Dunbar-Jacob, & Sereika's study

   b. Lewis & colleagues' study

   c. Bruce & Grove's study

6. What are the threats to external validity in:

   a. Berg, Dunbar-Jacob, & Sereika's study

   b. Lewis & colleagues' study

   c. Bruce & Grove's study

7. Identify three strengths in the design used by:

   a. Berg, Dunbar-Jacob, & Sereika_____

   _____

   _____

   b. Lewis and colleagues _____

   _____

   _____

   c. Bruce and Grove _____

   _____

   _____

⌘ GOING BEYOND

Examine the relationships among the study framework; research objectives, questions, or hypotheses; and design of the three studies in Appendix B.

1. Does the design allow an adequate test of the research objectives, questions, or hypotheses?
2. Does the design facilitate application of the findings to the framework?

References

Alsop-Shields, L. (1998). Changes in transcultural nursing and its influence on the growth of Australian Aboriginal children. *Journal of Pediatric Nursing, 13*(2), 119–126.

Anderson, K.M. (1998). Hypokalemic periodic paralysis: A case study. *American Journal of Critical Care, 7*(3), 236–239.

Bond, E.F., Heitkemper, M.M., & Jarrett, M. (1994). Intestinal transit and body weight responses to ovarian hormones and dietary fiber in rats. *Nursing Research, 43*(1), 18–24.

Burns, K.J., Camaione, D.N., Froman, R.D., & Clark, B.A. III. Predictors of referral to cardiac rehabilitation and cardiac exercise self-efficacy. *Clinical Nursing Research, 7*(2), 147–163.

Burns, S.M., Marshall, M., Burns, J.E., Ryan, B., Wilmoth, D., Carpenter, R., Aloi, A., Wood, M., & Truwit, J.D. (1998). Design, testing, and results of an outcomes-managed approach to patients requiring prolonged mechanical ventilation. *American Journal of Critical Care, 7*(1), 45–57.

Koshar, J.H., Lee, K.A., Goss, G., Heilemann, M.S., & Stinson, J. (1998). The Hispanic teen mother's origin of birth, use of prenatal care, and maternal and neonatal complications. *Journal of Pediatric Nursing, 13*(3), 151–157.

Medland, J.J., Ferrans, C.E., & the College of Nursing, University of Illinois at Chicago (1998). Effectiveness of a structured communication program for family members of patients in an ICU. *American Journal of Critical Care, 7*(1), 24–29.

Neville, K. (1998). The relationships among uncertainty, social support, and psychological distress in adolescents recently diagnosed with cancer. *Journal of Pediatric Oncology Nursing, 15*(1), 37–46.

Schrijvers, A.J.P. (1997). *Health and health care in The Netherlands. A critical self-assessment by Dutch experts in the medical and health sciences.* Utrecht: De Tijdstroom B.V.

Smeenk, F.W.J.M., de Witte, L.P., van Haastregt, J.C.M., Schipper, R.M., Biezemans, H.P.H., & Creboler, H.F.J.M. (1998). Transmural care of terminal cancer patients: Effects on the quality of life of direct caregivers. *Nursing Research, 47*(3), 129–136.

CHAPTER 8
POPULATIONS AND SAMPLES

⌘ INTRODUCTION

Read Chapter 8 and then complete the following exercises. These exercises will assist you in understanding the sampling process in published studies. The answers to these exercises are in Appendix A under Chapter 8.

⌘ RELEVANT TERMS

♦ **Directions:** Match each term with its correct definition.

a. accessible population
b. cluster sampling
c. convenience sampling
d. network sampling
e. nonprobability sampling
f. probability sampling
g. purposive sampling

h. quota sampling
i. random sampling
j. sampling
k. sampling criteria
l. stratified random sampling
m. systematic sampling
n. target population

Definitions

_____ 1. Process of selecting a group of people, events, behaviors, or other elements that are representative of the population being studied.
_____ 2. Portion of the target population to which the researcher has reasonable access.
_____ 3. All elements (people, objects, events, or substances) that meet the sample criteria for inclusion in a study.
_____ 4. Judgmental sampling that involves the conscious selection by the researcher of certain subjects or elements to include in a study.
_____ 5. List of the characteristics essential for membership in the target population.

____ 6. Random sampling technique in which every member (element) of the population has a probability higher than zero of being selected for the sample; examples include simple random sampling, stratified random sampling, cluster sampling, and systematic sampling.

____ 7. Sampling technique selecting every *k*th individual from an ordered list of all members of a population, using a randomly selected starting point.

____ 8. Random selection of elements from the sampling frame for inclusion in a study.

____ 9. Sampling technique used when the researcher knows some of the variables in the population that are critical to achieving representativeness; the sample is divided into strata or groups using these identified variables.

____ 10. Sampling technique in which a frame is developed that includes a list of all states, cities, institutions, or organizations that could be used in a study; a randomized sample is drawn from this list.

____ 11. Snowballing technique that takes advantage of social networks and the fact that friends tend to hold characteristics in common; subjects meeting sample criteria are asked to assist in locating others with similar characteristics.

____ 12. Sampling in which not every element of the population has an opportunity for selection, such as convenience sampling, quota sampling, purposive sampling, and network sampling.

____ 13. Convenience sampling technique with an added strategy to ensure the inclusion of subjects who are likely to be underrepresented in the convenience sample, such as women, minority groups, and uneducated people.

____ 14. Sampling technique that involves including subjects in a study because they happened to be in the right place at the right time.

⌘ KEY IDEAS

♦ **Directions:** Fill in the blanks with the appropriate word(s).

1. The individual units of a population are called _____.

2. The sample is obtained from the accessible population and is generalized to the

   _____.

3. *Representativeness* means that the _____,

   _____, and

   _____ are alike in as many ways as possible.

4. Identify two ways in which you might evaluate the representativeness of a sample in a published study.

   a. _____

   _____

   b. _____

   _____

5. Random variation is _____

   _____.

6. A list of every member of a population is referred to as a

   _____ .

7. A sampling plan outlines the _____

   _____ .

8. In critiquing the sampling plan in a study, what three things might you examine?

   a. _____

   b. _____

   c. _____

9. When the sampling criteria are narrowly defined or very specific, the sample desired is

   _____ .

10. When the sampling criteria are broadly defined to include a variety of subjects, the sample desired is _____ .

11. Subjects must be over the age of 18, able to read and write English, newly diagnosed with cancer, and have no other major illnesses. These are examples of

   _____ .

12. The sample was 65% female and 40% African American, 30% Hispanic, and 30% Caucasian; these are examples of _____ .

13. When subjects are lost to the study, this is referred to as _____ .

14. The term *control group* is limited to only those studies using

    _____ sampling methods.

15. If _____ sampling methods are used for sample selection,

    the group not receiving the treatment is referred to as a *comparison group*.

16. Identify four types of probability sampling.

    a. _____

    b. _____

    c. _____

    d. _____

17. When subjects are randomly assigned to treatment or control groups, this can be

    a _____ or _____

    sampling technique. If the original group of subjects is selected randomly prior to

    random assignment to treatment or control groups, it is considered a

    _____ sample.

18. Identify four types of nonprobability sampling.

    a. _____

    b. _____

    c. _____

    d. _____

19. Currently, do the majority of nursing studies use probability or nonprobability sampling

    methods? _____

20. Convenience sampling is also called _____.

21. Purposive sampling is referred to as _____.

22. The adequacy of the sample size can be evaluated using

    _____.

23. Power is the capacity to detect _____ or

    _____ that actually exist in the population.

24. The minimal acceptable level of power for a study is

    _____.

25. If the findings of a study are nonsignificant, the researcher should examine the adequacy

    of the sample size by running a _____.

26. Effect size is the extent to which the _____

    is false.

27. Identify five factors that influence the adequacy of a study's sample size.

    a. _____

       _____

    b. _____

       _____

    c. _____

       _____

    d. _____

       _____

    e. _____

       _____

⌘ MAKING CONNECTIONS

♦ **Directions:** Match the sampling method with the examples of sampling methods from published studies. Some of the sampling methods may be used more than once.

a. cluster sampling
b. convenience sampling
c. network sampling
d. purposive sampling
e. quota sampling

f. random assignment to groups
g. simple random sampling
h. stratified random sampling
i. systematic sampling

_____ 1. A sample of 500 nurses was randomly selected from a list of all registered nurses in the state of Texas.

_____ 2. A sample of 50 diabetic patients was obtained from an outpatient clinic and randomly placed in the comparison and experimental groups.

_____ 3. A sample of 10 HIV subjects was obtained by asking three subjects to identify their friends with HIV who might participate in the study.

_____ 4. A sample of 1000 critical care nurses was obtained by asking 100 critical care nurse managers in 50 randomly selected, large hospitals to identify 10 staff nurses to complete a survey.

_____ 5. A sample of 50 subjects was asked to participate in a study at an immunization booth in the mall.

_____ 6. Gender was used to stratify a sample of 100 randomly selected subjects.

_____ 7. The researcher obtained a list of all certified nurse practitioners, picked a random starting point, and then selected every 25th individual to participate in the study.

_____ 8. A sample of 50 hypertensive subjects was recruited in a clinic to participate in a study.

_____ 9. An equal number of patients with asthma, emphysema, and chronic bronchitis were recruited from the local Better Breathers Chapter to participate in a study.

_____ 10. The sample included 50 patients; 25 were examples of strong self-care and 25 were examples of poor self-care.

_____ 11. A sample of 5000 military personnel was randomly selected to participate in a study.

_____ 12. A sample of 10 drug-addicted nurses was obtained by asking five subjects to identify their friends who were drug-addicted.

_____ 13. Twenty-five home health patients were selected to participate in a study because they had a history of pressure ulcers that would not heal.

_____ 14. A sample of 50 adolescents was obtained at a fast food place.

_____ 15. A sample of 50 surgery patients was randomly selected from a hospital and randomly placed in control and treatment groups.

⌘ PUZZLES

Crossword Puzzle

♦ **Directions:** Complete the crossword puzzle using the clues on the following page. Note that if the answer is more than one word, there are no blank spaces left between words.

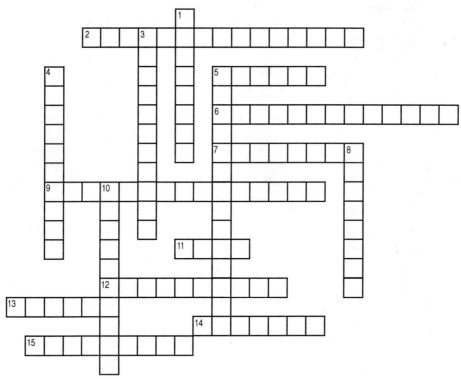

Across

2. group in a study
5. equal opportunity to be a subject
6. used to determine sample size
7. make up the population
9. used to select subjects
11. slanted from truth
12. portion of the target population within range of researcher
13. population designated by sample criteria
14. possible sampling method used when studying subjects with HIV
15. nonprobability sampling method

Down

1. determines who is in a sample
3. random sampling
4. number of subjects in a study
5. sample is _____ of population
8. people in a study
10. all members of a refined set

⌘ EXERCISES IN CRITIQUE

Bruce & Grove Study

♦ **Directions:** Review the Bruce & Grove (1994) article in Appendix B and answer the following questions.

1. List the sample criteria for this study.

2. Identify the sample characteristics for this study.

3. What is the sample size? _____ Was a power analysis used to determine the sample size?

4. Was the sample size adequate? Provide a rationale.

5. What was the sample mortality for this study? _____

6. Was probability or nonprobability sampling used in this study?

_____

7. What specific type of sampling method was used in this study?

_____

8. Was the sample in this study representative of the population studied? Provide a rationale.

9. Can the findings be generalized? Provide a rationale.

Berg, Dunbar-Jacob, & Sereika Study

♦ **Directions:** Review the Lewis & colleagues' study in Appendix B and answer the following questions.

1. List the sample criteria for this study.

2. Identify the sample characteristics for this study.

3. What is the sample size? _____ Describe the type of power analysis that was used to determine the sample size.

4. Was the sample size adequate? Provide a rationale.

5. What was the sample mortality for this study? _____

6. Was probability or nonprobability sampling used in this study?

   _____

7. What specific type of sampling method was used in this study?

   _____

8. Was the sample in this study representative of the population studied? Provide a rationale.

9. Can the findings be generalized? Provide a rationale.

Lewis & Colleagues' Study

♦ **Directions:** Review the Berg, Dunbar-Jacob, and Sereika article in Appendix B and answer the following questions.

1. List the sample criteria for this study.

2. Identify the sample characteristics for this study.

3. What is the sample size? _____ Was a power analysis used

   to determine the sample size? _____

4. Was the sample size adequate? Provide a rationale.

5. What was the sample mortality for this study? _____

6. Was probability or nonprobability sampling used in this study?

   _____

7. What specific type of sampling method was used in this study?

   _____

8. Was the sample in this study representative of the population studied? Provide a rationale.

9. Can the findings be generalized? Provide a rationale.

CHAPTER 9
MEASUREMENT AND DATA
COLLECTION IN RESEARCH

⌘ INTRODUCTION

Read Chapter 9 and then complete the following exercises. These exercises will assist you in learning relevant terms and identifying and critiquing measurement and data collection procedures in published studies. The answers to these exercises are in Appendix A under Chapter 9.

⌘ RELEVANT TERMS

♦ **Directions:** Define the following terms in your own words without looking at your textbook. Then check your definitions with those in the glossary of your textbook. Using this strategy, you can identify elements of the terms that are not yet clear in your mind. Reread the appropriate sections of the chapter to clarify your understanding of each term.

1. direct measurement _____

   _____

2. indirect measurement _____

   _____

3. instrumentation _____

   _____

4. nominal-scale measurement _____

   _____

5. ordinal-scale measurement _____

   _____

6. interval-scale measurement _____

   _____

7. measurement error _____

   _____

8. precision _____

   _____

9. accuracy _____

   _____

10. reliability _____

    _____

11. validity _____

    _____

⌘ KEY IDEAS

◆ **Directions:** Fill in the blanks with the appropriate word(s) or numbers.

1. The purpose of measurement is to produce _____ data.

2. The ideal, perfect measure is referred to as the _____
   measure.

3. Measurement _____ is the difference between true measure
   and what, in reality, is measured.

4. Weight is an example of _____ measurement.

5. A coping scale is an example of _____ measurement.

6. A reliability value of _____ is considered the lowest
   acceptable coefficient for a well-developed measurement tool.

Random Error

♦ **Directions:** Describe three measurement situations that might result in random error.

1. _____

   _____

   _____

2. _____

   _____

   _____

3. _____

   _____

   _____

Systematic Error

♦ **Directions:** Describe three measurement situations that might result in systematic error.

1. _____

   _____

   _____

2. _____

   _____

   _____

3. _____

   _____

   _____

Data Collection Tasks

♦ **Directions:** List five tasks of the researcher during data collection.

1. _____

2. _____

3. _____

4. _____

5. _____

⌘ MAKING CONNECTIONS

Measurement Error

♦ **Directions:** Match the type of measurement error likely to occur with the measurement method.

     a. random error

     b. systematic error

_____ 1. Community income using a white, middle-class sample

_____ 2. Severity of cancer at diagnosis in the community using patients in a county hospital

_____ 3. Average body weight measured at work at noon

_____ 4. Blood pressure taken with a stethoscope from which it is difficult to hear

_____ 5. Scores on a drug calculation test taken in a clinical setting any time during the work shift

Type of Reliability or Validity

♦ **Directions:** Match the type of reliability or validity with the definition.

_____ 1. test-retest reliability

_____ 2. interrater reliability

_____ 3. homogeneity

_____ 4. content validity

_____ 5. validity evidence from contrasting groups

_____ 6. validity evidence from examining convergence

_____ 7. validity evidence from examining divergence

_____ 8. validity evidence from discrimination analysis

_____ 9. validity evidence from predicting future events

_____ 10. validity evidence from predicting concurrent events

_____ 11. accuracy

_____ 12. precision

_____ 13. sensitivity

a. comparison of values with those of other instruments that measure the same concept

b. amount of change that can be measured

c. comparison of values with those of other instruments that measure similar concepts

d. consistency of measurement of two raters

e. comparison of groups expected to have opposing responses to instrument items

f. adequacy of operational definition

g. evaluates consistency of repeated measures

h. comparison of values with those of other instruments that measure opposite concepts

i. ability of instrument values to predict future performance

j. ability to predict current value of measure based on value from measure of another concept

k. correlation of various items within an instrument

l. consistency of measurement

m. extent to which all elements of a concept are measured

⌘ PUZZLES

Word Scramble

Rethe si on fertpec semarue.

Secret Message

Anurjkrurch cnbcrwp bqxdum kn ynaoxavnm xw njlq rwbcadvnwc dbnm rw j bcdmh.

Crossword Puzzle

♦ **Directions:** Complete the crossword puzzle. Note that if the answer is more than one word, there are no blank spaces left between words.

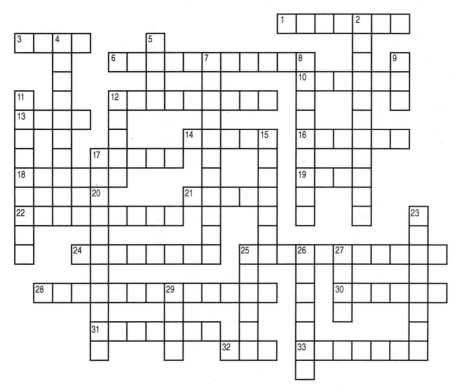

Across

1. gather data
3. most common method of obtaining questionnaire data
6. strategies used to produce trustworthy data
10. the crudest form of scale
12. concerned with the consistency of repeated measures
13. infrequent occurrence
14. highest level of measurement
16. self-report measures with summated scores
17. the difference between true measure and what is measured
18. used for observation
19. unstructured
21. site of data collection

22. measurement strategy involving verbal communication between the researcher and the subject
24. evaluation of the adequacy of a physiologic operational definition
25. the amount of change of a parameter that can be measured precisely
28. a printed self-report form with individual items that are not summated
30. scale with options rated from negative to positive
31. level of measurement in which values must be ranked
32. common method of obtaining demographic data
33. lowest level of measurement

Down

2. interrater reliability
4. a measurement device
5. information obtained through measurement
7. consistency of measurement
8. the perfect measurement
9. commonly used demographic data
11. references subjects' score to target behaviors
12. value obtained from measurement
15. most subjective form of measurement

20. approach to judging accuracy of physiologic measures
23. level of measurement with equal numerical distances
25. commonly measured concept
26. place in which data collection occurs
27. common source of observational data
29. last single-digit value

⌘ EXERCISES IN CRITIQUE

♦ **Directions:** Review the research articles in Appendix B and answer the following questions.

1. Using the following table, identify the variables measured, the method of measurement, and the directness of measurement (D = direct, I = indirect).

Berg, Dunbar-Jacob, & Sereika's study

Variable	Method of Measurement	Directness

Lewis & colleagues' study

Variable	Method of Measurement	Directness

Bruce & Grove's study

Variable	Method of Measurement	Directness

2. Critique the thoroughness with which each method of measurement was described. In
   making this judgment, look for the following information about the measurement
   method: (a) developer of the method of measurement; (b) date measurement method was
   developed; (c) detailed description of method of measurement (*i.e.,* number of items in
   scale, steps of performing a physiologic measure); (d) range of values possible using the
   measure.

   Berg, Dunbar-Jacob, & Sereika's study

   a. Measure _____

   b. Measure _____

c. Measure _____

d. Measure _____

e. Measure _____

Lewis & colleagues' study

a. Measure _____

Bruce & Grove's study

a. Measure _____

b. Measure _____

c. Measure _____

d. Measure _____

3. To examine the reliability and validity of each measure, identify the types of reliability and validity reported for each measure and the numerical values reported for each using the following table. Of particular interest is whether reliability was examined in the sample used in the study.

Berg, Dunbar-Jacob, & Sereika's study

Measure _____

Type of Reliability or Validity	Value	From Present Sample?

Measure _____

Type of Reliability or Validity	Value	From Present Sample?

Measure _____

Type of Reliability or Validity	Value	From Present Sample?

Measure _____

Type of Reliability or Validity	Value	From Present Sample?

Measure _____

Type of Reliability or Validity	Value	From Present Sample?

Lewis and colleagues' study

Measure _____

Type of Reliability or Validity	Value	From Present Sample?

Bruce and Grove's study

Measure _____

Type of Reliability or Validity	Value	From Present Sample?

Measure _____

Type of Reliability or Validity	Value	From Present Sample?

Measure _____

Type of Reliability or Validity	Value	From Present Sample?

Measure _____

Type of Reliability or Validity	Value	From Present Sample?

4. In each study, look for a description of the data collection process. Look for inconsistencies in measurements. Identify threats to the validity of the measures.
   a. Berg, Dunbar-Jacob, & Sereika's study

   b. Lewis & colleagues' study

   c. Bruce & Grove's study

5. Using the information gathered above, judge the adequacy of each measure used in each study.
   a. Berg, Dunbar-Jacob, & Sereika's study

   b. Lewis & colleagues' study

    c. Bruce & Grove's study

⌘ GOING BEYOND

Identify a quasi-experimental study in a recent nursing journal. Identify the intervention or treatment. Was the intervention described in sufficient detail for you to provide the same intervention? Was the intervention provided consistently to all subjects? In your opinion, was the intervention sufficiently powerful to cause a difference in the effect between the experimental and control groups? Write a brief paragraph judging the adequacy of the intervention.

CHAPTER 10
UNDERSTANDING STATISTICS
IN RESEARCH

⌘ INTRODUCTION

Read Chapter 10 and then complete the following exercises. These exercises will assist you in learning relevant terms and identifying and critiquing statistics in published studies. The answers to these exercises are in Appendix A under Chapter 10.

⌘ RELEVANT TERMS

♦ **Directions:** Define the following terms in your own words without looking at your textbook. Then check your definitions with those in the glossary of your textbook. Using this strategy, you can identify elements of the terms that are not yet clear in your mind. Reread the appropriate sections of the chapter to clarify your understanding of each term.

1. central tendency _____

   _____

2. clinical significance _____

   _____

3. dependent groups _____

   _____

4. variance _____

   _____

5. distribution _____

   _____

6. frequencies _____

_____

7. generalization _____

_____

8. inference _____

_____

9. outliers _____

_____

10. power _____

_____

11. relationship _____

_____

12. statistic _____

_____

13. tailedness _____

_____

⌘ KEY IDEAS

♦ **Directions:** Fill in the blanks with the appropriate word(s) or numbers.

1. List four activities of data cleaning.

    a. _____

    b. _____

    c. _____

    d. _____

2. List three statistical strategies used to describe the sample.

    a. _____

    b. _____

    c. _____

⌘ MAKING CONNECTIONS

♦ **Directions:** Perform the following matching exercises.

Matching Definitions

_____ 1. exploratory analysis

_____ 2. outliers

_____ 3. probability

_____ 4. inference

_____ 5. generalization

_____ 6. type I error

_____ 7. type II error

_____ 8. power

_____ 9. decision theory

a. accepts null hypothesis when it is false

b. the probability that a statistical test will detect a significant difference that exists

c. conclusion based on evidence

d. information applied to population that has been acquired from a specific instance

e. rejects null hypothesis when it is true

f. the likelihood of an event occurring in a given situation

g. assumption of no difference

h. subjects with extreme values

i. descriptive examination of the data

Matching Categories to Statements

a. decision theory statement

b. probability theory statement

c. inference

d. generalization

_____ 1. As hypothesized, the experimental systematic nursing assessment successfully forestalled the increase in symptom distress (Sarna, 1998, p. 1044).

_____ 2. This suggests that when psychological distress occurs, disruption in sexual activity and sexual desire also are likely to be present (Steginga, Occhipinti, Wilson, & Dunn, 1998, p. 1068).

_____ 3. No significant differences in functional and psychosocial outcomes were found between the two groups of patients treated with AMP [amputation] or LS [limb-sparing] surgical procedure (Hudson, Tyc, Cremer, Luo, Li, Rao, Meyer, Crom, & Pratt, 1998, p. 68).

_____ 4. Because most major risk factors thought to affect skin health did not change (*i.e.,* body movement, skin moisture, fecal incontinence frequency) and no adverse changes in skin health were observed during the intervention period, it is plausible to argue that the individualized intervention would not have adverse skin effects if applied over longer time periods (Schnelle, Criuse, Alessi, Al-Samarrai, & Ouslander, 1998, p. 203).

_____ 5. The results of this study indicate that GBI [geragogy-based instruction] can aid in increasing medication knowledge in a rural elderly ED [emergency department] population. Written medication instructions that are large print, on a fourth to fifth grade reading level, and organized in the elderly schema for remembering medications appear to be successful in the teaching and learning of medication information (Hayes, 1998, p. 216).

_____ 6. The results of the path analysis provided empirical support for the theoretical model of the direct and indirect effects of perceived self-efficacy on depressive symptoms (Kurlowicz, 1998, p. 223).

_____ 7. Automatic cuffs can be used safely for frequent assessment of blood pressure in patients with acute myocardial infarction who are receiving thrombolytic therapy (Saul, Smith, & Mook, 1998, p. 195).

Significant Differences

In testing for significant differences between groups, the researcher is determining whether the experimental group belongs to the same population as the control group. An initial step in this process is to compare the mean and standard deviation of the control group with those of the experimental group. The normal curve can be used to visually depict differences in these measures between the two groups. For example, Maloni, Chance, Zhang, Cohen, Betts, and Gange (1993) compared the physical and psychosocial side effects of antepartum hospital complete bed rest, partial bed rest, and no bed rest. Using the no-bed-rest group as the control group, we can compare these three groups. For the variable of weight gain, the no-bed-rest group mean (M) was 14.48 with a standard deviation (SD) of 4.94. Using this information, the distribution of weight gain in the no-bed-rest group can be illustrated.

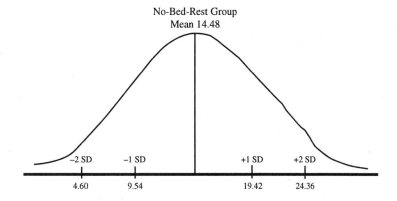

No-Bed-Rest Group
Mean 14.48

−2 SD −1 SD +1 SD +2 SD
4.60   9.54   19.42 24.36

The mean for the partial-bed-rest group was 10.90 with a standard deviation of 5.29. Using the following curve, illustrate the distribution of values as shown on the previous page.

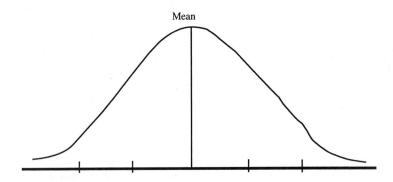

The mean for the complete-bed-rest group was 8.17 with a standard deviation of 2.09. Using the following curve, illustrate the distribution of values.

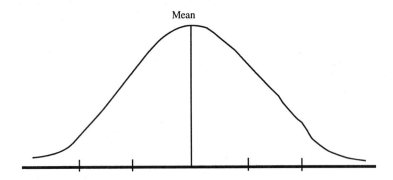

Statistical analyses are required to determine if the differences in weight gain in the three groups indicates that the groups represent different populations. ANOVA results were F = 7.79 with df = 2,28 and p = .002 indicating that the groups are significantly different.

Significance of Results

♦ **Directions:** In the following statistical reports, indicate whether the results were significant, assuming a level of significance set at .05.

    a. significant
    b. not significant

_____ 1. The study examined psychosocial adjustment of males to three types of dialysis. ANOVA was used to examine differences among the three dialysis types. The results were as follows: $F = 4$, $df = 2$, $p < .0467$ (Courts & Boyette, 1998, p. 54).

_____ 2. The study examined the safety of automatic versus manual blood pressure cuffs for patients receiving thrombolytic therapy. Purpura developed in 33 subjects (34%), 17 of whom had blood pressure measured with a manual cuff and 16 of whom had blood pressure measured with an automatic device ($p = .883$) (Saul, Smith, & Mook, 1998).

_____ 3. The study examined the relationship between psychological distress and gastrointestinal symptoms in women with irritable bowel syndrome. There was a significant positive relationship between the Turmoil score [measuring psychological distress] and GI Distress score, $\beta = 0.47$, SE of $\beta = 0.11$, $t(96) = 4.30$, $p < .001$ (Jarrett, Heitkempter, Cain, Tuftin, Walker, Bond, & Levy, 1998, p. 159).

_____ 4. The study examined moderators of the relationship between trait anxiety and information received by patients post-myocardial infarction. When information received was regressed on the product of trait anxiety and gender, the beta was $-.10$ ($p = .42$) and the R^2 change was .009, $F = .66$, $p = .42$ (Yarcheski, Proctor, & Oriscello, 1998).

⌘ PUZZLES

Word Scramble

To eb fuelus, het decineve morf taad yalinass stum eb lulefarcy maxidene, groznadie, dan venig ginneam.

Secret Message

Viwievglivw ger riziv tvszi xlmrkw.

Crossword Puzzle

♦ **Directions:** Complete the crossword puzzle. Note that if the answer is more than one word, there are no blank spaces left between words.

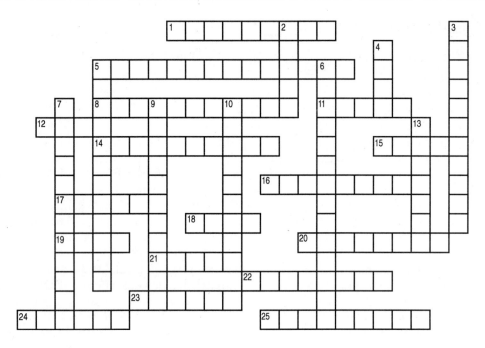

Across

1. a numerical value obtained from a sample
5. uses cut-off point to judge significance of differences
8. unlikely that results are due to chance
11. probability that an analysis will detect a difference that exists
12. exclude incomplete data from analysis
14. analysis used to predict the value of one variable if values of other variables are known
15. test that uses variance to compare differences between groups
16. groups in which subjects are related to selection of other subjects
17. determines an outcome
18. measure of central tendency for interval data
19. extreme of the normal curve
20. dispersion of values in sample
21. difference between lowest value and highest value

22. subjects with extreme values unlike the rest of the sample
23. measure of central tendency for ordinal data
24. outcome of data analysis
25. judgment based on evidence

Down

2. analysis technique used to determine differences between two samples
3. statistical procedures used to examine the data descriptively
4. measure of central tendency for nominal data
5. the dispersion of values
6. sample that is like the population
7. meanings of conclusions for the body of nursing knowledge
9. theoretical symmetrical distribution of all possible values
10. statistical test used to analyze nominal data
13. statistical tests developed to determine location of differences after ANOVA

⌘ EXERCISES IN CRITIQUE

♦ **Directions:** Refer to Bruce & Grove's study in Appendix B and answer the following questions. The research question for Bruce & Grove's study is: What is the difference in the mean total serum cholesterol, LDL cholesterol, and HDL cholesterol and cardiovascular risk levels of military members before and after participation in the C.A.R.E. program?

1. List the variables that will be used in statistical analyses to answer this question and the level of measurement of each variable.

Variable	Level of Measurement

2. Bruce & Grove chose to conduct two separate statistical analyses to answer their research question using the variables listed above. What were these statistical procedures?
   a.

   b.

3. Identify the groups used in the first analysis described in their research paper.
   a.

   b.

4. Were these two groups independent or dependent?

5. Using the algorithm on page 328 in your textbook, judge the appropriateness of the statistical procedure used for the analysis. Can you identify other statistical procedures that might have been better? Write a brief paragraph expressing your judgment.

6. One variable was excluded from the first analysis. What was this variable?

7. Why was this variable excluded? (Use the information from questions A and B. In your textbook, reread the discussion on the statistical procedure selected for this analysis.)

8. State the results of the analysis, providing numerical values. Circle the appropriate categorization of the results.

   a. significant and predicted
   b. nonsignificant
   c. significant and not predicted
   d. mixed results
   e. unexpected

9. Identify the groups used in the second analysis described in Bruce & Grove's research paper.
   a.

   b.

   c.

   d.

   e.

10. Using the algorithm on page 328 in your textbook, judge the appropriateness of the statistical procedure used for the analysis. Can you identify other statistical procedures that might have been better? Write a brief paragraph expressing your judgment.

11. State the results of the analysis, providing numerical values. Circle the appropriate categorization of the results.

   a. significant and predicted
   b. nonsignificant
   c. significant and not predicted
   d. mixed results
   e. unexpected

12. A third statistical procedure was performed that was not necessary to answer the research question but provided additional information about the variables. What was this procedure?

13. Identify the variables included in each of the three analyses and the results. Indicate whether each result was significant and predicted, nonsignificant, significant and not predicted, mixed, or unexpected.
   a.

   b.

   c.

14. Identify the findings reported by the authors. Compare these findings to the results you have just examined. Judge the appropriateness of the findings in relation to the results. Write a short paragraph giving your evaluation of the linkage between the results and the findings.

15. Write a brief paragraph discussing the strengths and weaknesses of the analysis strategies used in the study.

16. Identify conclusions made by the authors based on their findings.

17. Write a brief paragraph judging whether the conclusions are warranted by the data.

18. Identify the implications made by the authors.

19. Write a brief paragraph evaluating these implications. Include implications you were able to identify that were not considered by the authors.

20. Write a brief paragraph assessing the clinical significance of these findings.

21. Were the findings generalized? If so, to what populations? List the populations.

22. What suggestions did the authors make for further studies? List the studies they suggested.

⌘ GOING BEYOND

Perform a similar critique of the analyses used by Berg, Dunbar-Jacob, & Sereika and by Lewis & colleagues.

References

Courts, N.F., & Boyette, B.G. (1998). Psychosocial adjustment of males on three types of dialysis. *Clinical Nursing Research, 7*(1), 47–63.

Fawcett, J., Pollio, N., Tully, A., Barron, M., Henklein, J.C., & Jones, R.C. (1993). Effects of information on adaptation to cesarean birth. *Nursing Research, 42*(1), 49–53.

Griffith, P., James, B., & Cropp, A. (1994). Evaluation of the safety and efficacy of topical nitroglycerin ointment to facilitate venous cannulation. *Nursing Research, 43*(4), 203–206.

Hayes, K. (1998). Randomized trial of geregogy-based medication instruction in the emergency department. *Nursing Research, 47*(4), 211–218.

Hudson, M.M., Tyc, V.L., Cremer, L.K., Luo, X., Rao, B.N., Meyer, W.H.,, Crom, D.B., & Pratt, C.B. (1998). Patient satisfaction after limb-sparing surgery and amputation for pediatric malignant bone tumors. *Journal of Pediatric Oncology Nursing, 15*(2), 60–69.

Kurlowicz, L.H. (1998). Perceived self-efficacy, functional ability, and depressive symptoms in older elective surgery patients. *Nursing Research, 47*(4), 219–226.

Maloni, J.A., Chance, B., Zhang, C., Cohen, A.W., Betts, D., & Gange, S.J. (1993). Physical and psychosocial side effects of antepartum hospital bed rest. *Nursing Research, 42*(4), 197–203.

Metheny, N., Reed, L., Wiersema, L., McSweeney, M., Wehrle, M.A., & Clark, J. (1993). Effectiveness of pH measurements in predicting feeding tube placement: An update. *Nursing Research, 42*(6), 324–331.

O'Brien, M.T. (1993). Multiple sclerosis: The relationship among self-esteem, social support, and coping behavior. *Applied Nursing Research, 6*(2), 54–63.

Sarna, L. (1998). Effectiveness of structured nursing assessment of symptom distress in advanced lung cancer. *Oncology Nursing Forum, 25*(6), 1041–1048.

Sarna, L., Smith, J., & Mook, W. (1998). The safety of automatic versus manual blood pressure cuffs for patients receiving thrombolytic therapy. *American Journal of Critical Care, 7*(3), 192–196.

Schnelle, J.F., Criuse, P.A., Alessi, C.A., Al-Samarrai, N., & Ouslander, J.G. (1998). Individualizing nighttime incontinence care in nursing home residents. *Nursing Research, 47*(4), 197–204.

Shoaf, J., & Oliver, S. (1992). Efficacy of normal saline injection with and without heparin for maintaining intermittent intravenous site. *Applied Nursing Research, 5*(1), 9–12.

Wakefield, B., Wakefield, D.S., & Booth, B.M. (1992). Evaluating the validity of blood glucose monitoring strip interpretation by experienced users. *Applied Nursing Research, 5*(1), 13–19.

CHAPTER 11
INTRODUCTION TO
QUALITATIVE RESEARCH

⌘ INTRODUCTION

Read Chapter 11 and then complete the following exercises. These exercises will assist you in learning relevant terms and reading and comprehending published qualitative studies. The answers to these exercises are in Appendix A under Chapter 11.

⌘ RELEVANT TERMS

♦ **Directions:** Define the following terms in your own words without looking at your textbook. Then check your definitions with those in the glossary of your textbook. Using this strategy, you can identify elements of the terms that are not yet clear in your mind. Reread the appropriate sections of the chapter to clarify your understanding of each term.

1. decision trail _____

   _____

2. holistic _____

   _____

3. reductionism _____

   _____

4. reflexive thought _____

   _____

5. rigor _____

   _____

⌘ MAKING CONNECTIONS

♦ **Directions:** Match the characteristic with the type of research.

     a. qualitative
     b. quantitative

____ 1. produces "hard" science
____ 2. philosophical approach to research
____ 3. truth is absolute
____ 4. reductionistic
____ 5. holistic
____ 6. researcher remains objective and detached
____ 7. truth is dynamic
____ 8. control is important
____ 9. subjectivity is essential
____ 10. unstructured

⌘ KEY IDEAS

♦ **Directions:** Fill in the blanks with the correct responses.

1. List three characteristics of rigor in qualitative studies.

    a. _____

    b. _____

    c. _____

2. List three characteristics of researcher-participant relationships in qualitative research.

    a. _____

    b. _____

    c. _____

3. List four methods of reducing data in qualitative research.

   a. _____

   b. _____

   c. _____

   d. _____

4. List three data collection methods commonly used in qualitative studies.

   a. _____

   b. _____

   c. _____

5. List three stages of qualitative data analysis.

   a. _____

   b. _____

   c. _____

♦ **Directions:** Fill in the blanks with the correct responses.

      a. phenomenological
      b. grounded theory
      c. ethnographic
      d. historical

_____ 1. studies cultures

_____ 2. studies interactions of individuals or groups

_____ 3. studies the meaning of a lived experience

_____ 4. uses informants

_____ 5. used by Benner to examine clinical practice

_____ 6. studies the past

_____ 7. gaining entry is essential

_____ 8. uses a constant comparative process

_____ 9. develops an inventory of sources

_____ 10. considers an experience unique to the individual

Storytelling Exercise

1. Tape record a story told to you by a friend or family member. Write the story in step-by-step narrative form. Include the following information.
   a. What is this about?
   b. Who? What? When? Where?
   c. Then what happened?
   d. So what?
   e. What finally happened?
   f. Finish the narrative.
2. What is the purpose of the story?
   a. make a point
   b. be moralistic
   c. a success story
   d. a reminder of what not to do or how not to be
   e. guidance in how to avoid the fate described in the story

⌘ GOING BEYOND

Select a qualitative study from a recent nursing journal.

1. Identify the type of qualitative study performed.
2. Identify the data collection methods used.
3. What were the relationships between the researcher and participants?
4. Identify the following steps of data analysis:
   a. description
   b. analysis
   c. interpretation
5. Evaluate the rigor of the study.
6. Do the authors address a decision trail?

CHAPTER 12
CRITIQUING NURSING STUDIES

⌘ INTRODUCTION

Read Chapter 12 and then complete the following exercises. These exercises will assist you in understanding the quantitative and qualitative research critique processes. The answers to these exercises are in Appendix A under Chapter 12.

⌘ RELEVANT TERMS

♦ **Directions:** Match each term with its correct definition.

a. analysis step of critique
b. analytic preciseness
c. auditability
d. comparison step of critique
e. comprehension step of critique

f. descriptive vividness
g. evaluation step of critique
h. heuristic relevance
i. methodological congruence
j. theoretical connectedness

_____ 1. Standard for evaluating qualitative research, in which documentation rigor, procedural rigor, ethical rigor, and auditability of the study are examined.

_____ 2. Rigorous development of a decision trail that is reported in sufficient detail to allow a second researcher to use the original data and the decision trail to arrive at conclusions similar to those of the original researcher.

_____ 3. Critique step that involves determining the strengths and limitations of the logical links connecting one study element with another.

_____ 4. Theoretical schema developed from a qualitative study; the schema is clearly expressed, logically consistent, reflective of the data, and compatible with nursing's knowledge base.

_____ 5. Critique step in which the reader examines the meaning and significance of a study according to set criteria and compares it with previous studies conducted in the area.

_____ 6. Performing a series of transformations during which concrete data are transformed across several levels of abstractions to develop a theoretical schema that imparts meaning to the phenomenon under study.

_____ 7. Critique step during which the reader gains understanding of the terms in the research report; identifies the study elements; and grasps the nature, significance, and meaning of these elements.

_____ 8. Standard for evaluating a qualitative study, in which the study's intuitive recognition, relationship to the existing body of knowledge, and applicability are examined.

_____ 9. Description of the site, subjects, experience of collecting data, and the researcher's thoughts during the qualitative research process are presented clearly enough that the reader has the sense of personally experiencing the event.

_____ 10. Critique step in which the ideal for each step of the quantitative research process is compared with the real steps in a published study.

⌘ KEY IDEAS

♦ **Directions:** Fill in the blanks with the appropriate word(s).

1. An intellectual research critique involves careful examination of all aspects of a study to

   judge the _____, _____,

   _____, and _____ of the study.

2. Identify three important questions that are part of an intellectual research critique.

   a. _____

   b. _____

   c. _____

3. Describe your role in conducting research critiques.

4. List the four steps of the quantitative research critique process.

   a. _____

   b. _____

   c. _____

   d. _____

5. Identify the five standards used to critique qualitative studies.

   a. _____

   b. _____

   c. _____

   d. _____

   e. _____

⌘ EXERCISES IN CRITIQUE

◆ **Directions:** Read the research articles in Appendix B. Conduct the steps of the quantitative research critique process (comprehension, comparison, analysis, and evaluation) on these three studies using the guidelines in Chapter 12 of your textbook. Many parts of these studies were critiqued in Chapters 3–10 of this study guide.

For each study, perform the following steps:

   a. Conduct the comprehension step of the critique process. Questions are outlined in your text to direct your critique.
   b. Do a critique that includes the comparison, analysis, and evaluation steps of the quantitative research critique process.

1. Berg, Dunbar-Jacob, & Sereika (1997)

2. Lewis & colleagues (1997)

3. Bruce & Grove (1994)

CHAPTER 13
USING RESEARCH IN
NURSING PRACTICE

⌘ INTRODUCTION

Read Chapter 13 and then complete the following exercises. These exercises will assist you in understanding the process for using research findings in practice. The answers to these exercises are in Appendix A under Chapter 13.

⌘ RELEVANT TERMS

♦ **Directions:** Match each term with the correct definitions and descriptions.

    a. communication of research findings
    b. Conduct and Utilization of Research in Nursing (CURN) project
    c. innovation
    d. innovators
    e. meta-analysis
    f. research utilization
    g. Rogers' Innovation-Decision Process
    h. Western Interstate Commission for Higher Education (WICHE) regional nursing research development project

_____ 1. The use of statistical analysis and the interpretation of the results to merge the findings from several studies to determine what is known about a particular phenomenon.

_____ 2. Process that includes the steps of knowledge, persuasion, decision, implementation, and confirmation to promote diffusion or communication of research findings to members of a discipline.

_____ 3. Process by which research knowledge is communicated to members of a social system to achieve a desired outcome.

_____ 4. Developing a research report and disseminating it through presentations and publications to practicing nurses, other health professionals, consumers, and policy makers.

_____ 5. Idea, practice, or object that is perceived as new by a person, a nursing unit, an entire agency, or other decision-making unit.

_____ 6. First major research utilization project in nursing that involved the collaboration of clinicians and educators in critiquing studies and developing detailed plans for using selected research findings in practice.

_____ 7. People who actively seek out new ideas.

_____ 8. The purpose of this project was to increase the use of research findings in practice by communicating the findings, facilitating organizational modifications necessary for implementation, and encouraging collaborative research that is directly useful in clinical practice.

⌘ KEY IDEAS

♦ **Directions:** Fill in the blanks with the appropriate word(s).

1. List four reasons why nurses need to use research findings in practice.

   a. _____

   b. _____

   c. _____

   d. _____

2. Think about the clinical agency where you are currently doing your clinical hours.

   a. Are the agencies' policies and nursing protocols based on research?

   b. What is the basis of the policies and protocols if it is not research?

   c. Who are the innovators in this agency? Record only the names of the people's positions.

    d. Who might be resistant to change?

    e. Does the agency provide research publications for nurses? List some examples of
       these publications.

3. Identify three sources that you might access to keep current with the research literature.

    a. _____

    b. _____

    c. _____

4. Identify two reports that were published from the WICHE project.

    a. _____

    b. _____

5. Identify the four-step research utilization process used in the CURN project.

    a. _____

    b. _____

    c. _____

    d. _____

6. Identify six topics in which research findings were considered worthy of implementation
   in practice in the CURN project.

    a. _____

    b. _____

    c. _____

    d. _____

    e. _____

    f. _____

7. Identify the three types of barriers to using research findings in nursing practice and provide an example of each.

   a. _____

      Example _____

   b. _____

      Example _____

   c. _____

      Example _____

8. Identify three prior conditions of an agency that need to be examined when planning to make a change based on research.

   a. _____

   b. _____

   c. _____

9. Identify the five characteristics of the innovation or change in practice that need to be examined during the persuasion stage.

   a. _____

   b. _____

   c. _____

   d. _____

   e. _____

10. Active rejection of a change in practice involves _____

    _____

11. Passive rejection of a change in practice indicates _____

    _____

12. Identify and describe the three ways in which research findings might be implemented in nursing practice.

a. _____ Description _____

_____

b. _____ Description _____

_____

c. _____ Description _____

_____

13. During the confirmation stage, discontinuance of the change in practice can occur. What are the two types of discontinuance?

   a. _____

   b. _____

14. Identify two sources of summaries of nursing research knowledge.

   a. _____

   b. _____

⌘ MAKING CONNECTIONS

◆ **Directions:** Match the stage in Rogers' Innovation–Decision Process with the appropriate description.

   a. knowledge   d. implementation
   b. persuasion   e. confirmation
   c. decision

____ 1. The stage at which the nurses evaluate the effectiveness of the change in practice and decide to either continue or discontinue it.
____ 2. The stage at which the innovation is either adopted or rejected.
____ 3. The first awareness of the existence of an innovation or new idea for use in practice.
____ 4. The stage at which the innovation or change is put to use by a person, unit, or agency.
____ 5. The stage at which a person or agency develops a favorable or unfavorable attitude toward the change or innovation.

⌘ GOING BEYOND

Conduct a project to use research findings in practice. Use the content and example of research utilization in Chapter 13 and the following steps as a guide.

1. Identify a clinical problem that might be improved by using research knowledge.
2. Locate and review the studies in this problem area.
3. Summarize what is known and not known regarding this problem. (See Chapter 3 for additional direction in summarizing research literature.)
4. Select a model or theory to direct your use of research findings in practice, such as Rogers' Innovation–Decision Process.
5. Assess your agency's readiness to make the change (prior conditions in Rogers' Model, presented on p. 431 of your text).
6. Persuade the nursing personnel, other health professionals, and administration to make the change in practice. This is the Persuasion Stage of Rogers' Model.
7. Have those people involved in the change make a decision to adopt or reject the change (Rogers' Implementation Stage).
8. Implement the change by developing a protocol or policy that clearly indicates the change needed for practice. Communicate this protocol or policy to members of the clinical agency (Rogers' Implementation Stage).
9. Develop evaluation strategies to determine the effect of the change. You might examine cost, patient outcomes, and nursing workload (Rogers' Confirmation Stage).
10. Evaluate over time to determine if the change continued. You might also extend the change to additional units or clinical agencies.

APPENDIX A

ANSWERS TO STUDY
GUIDE EXERCISES

CHAPTER 1
DISCOVERING NURSING RESEARCH

RELEVANT TERMS

1. f
2. g
3. a
4. d
5. i
6. l
7. b
8. o

9. e
10. n
11. k
12. c
13. h
14. m
15. j

KEY IDEAS

1. **Description** involves identifying the nature and attributes of nursing phenomena. Descriptive knowledge generated through research can be used to identify what exists in nursing practice, discover new information, and classify information of use in the discipline. Examples include describing those who are at risk for HIV or identifying the symptoms for making a nursing diagnosis.
2. **Explanation** focuses on clarifying relationships among variables or identifying reasons why certain events occur. For example, risk of developing pressure ulcers is related to level of mobility and age; as mobility decreases and age increases, pressure ulcer risk increases.
3. **Prediction** involves estimating the probability of a specific outcome in a given situation. With predictive knowledge, nurses can anticipate the effects nursing interventions might have on patients and families. For example, they might predict the effects of a long-term exercise program on women with breast cancer.
4. **Control** is the ability to manipulate a situation to produce the desired outcome. Nurses prescribe certain interventions to help patients and families achieve quality outcomes. For example, you would prescribe the use of warm, not cold, applications for the resolution of normal saline IV infiltrations.

Historical Events Influencing Nursing Research

1. Nightingale
2. 1952
3. ANA Council of Nurse Researchers
4. research
5. *Research in Nursing & Health*
6. *Western Journal of Nursing Research*

7. *Scholarly Inquiry for Nursing Practice*
   Applied Nursing Research
   Nursing Science Quarterly
8. Conduct and Utilization of Research in Nursing (CURN)
9. summaries of current research knowledge in the areas of nursing practice, nursing care delivery, nursing education, and the nursing profession.
10. 1985
11. National Institute for Nursing Research (NINR)
12. conducting, supporting, disseminating information
13. You could have identified any four of the following:
    a. effectiveness of nursing interventions in HIV/AIDS
    b. cognitive impairment
    c. community-based nursing models
    d. living with chronic illness
    e. behavior factors related to immunocompetence
14. clinical
15. Agency for Health Care Policy and Research (AHCPR)
16. scientific or empirical

Acquiring Knowledge in Nursing

1. You could have identified any seven of the following ways of acquiring knowledge in nursing. Some possible examples of each way of acquiring nursing knowledge are provided.
   a. tradition: giving report on hospitalized patients in a specific way or organizing the care provided to the patients in a specific, structured way.
   b. authority: expert nurses, educators, and authors of articles or books.
   c. borrowing: using knowledge from medicine or psychology in nursing practice
   d. trial and error: positioning a patient to reduce his or her discomfort
   e. personal experience: obtaining knowledge by being in a clinical agency and providing care to patients and families
   f. role-modeling: a new graduate in an internship is mentored by an expert nurse
   g. intuition: knowing that a patient's condition is deteriorating but having no concrete data to support this feeling or hunch
   h. reasoning: reasoning from the general to the specific or deductive reasoning. Reasoning from the specific to the general or inductive reasoning.
   i. research: quantitative, qualitative, and outcomes research methods
2. personal experience
3. novice, advanced beginner, competent, proficient, and expert
4. borrowed
5. research, empirical, or scientific
6. intuition
7. traditions
8. mentorship relationship
9. role-model

10. inductive, deductive
11. deductive reasoning
12. quantitative, qualitative, outcomes
13. outcomes research
14. Identify common interventions used in practice, such as taking a temperature, providing oral care, treating an ulcer, changing a dressing on a wound. Use the content in your textbook to determine the knowledge base for each of the interventions you identified. Nursing knowledge is acquired through tradition, authority, borrowing, trial and error, personal experience, role-modeling, intuition, reasoning, and research.
15. Examine the interventions you use in clinical practice and decide which way of acquiring knowledge you use most frequently: tradition, authority, borrowing, trial and error, personal experience, role-modeling, intuition, reasoning, or research.
16. Important outcomes include outcomes such as patient health status (signs, symptoms, functional status, morbidity, mortality), patient satisfaction, costs related to health care, quality of care, and quality of care provider.

MAKING CONNECTIONS

Types of Research Methods

1. b   5. a
2. b   6. a
3. a   7. a
4. b   8. b

Nurses' Educational Preparation

1. a   5. b
2. e   6. c
3. b   7. d
4. d

PUZZLES

Word Scramble

1. Both quantitative and qualitative research are essential to develop nursing knowledge.
2. Research knowledge is needed to control outcomes in nursing practice.

EXERCISES IN CRITIQUE

1. c
2. c
3. c
1. Berg has a PhD and had obtained funding for this study from two sources. Dunbar-Jacob has a PhD and has conducted funded research in the area of chronic disorders. Sereika has a PhD and a strong background in biostatistics and epidemiology. These people have very strong research preparation for conducting this study in addition to the funding.

2. Liehr is PhD-prepared and employed by the University of Texas Health Science Center in Houston. Lewis, Mackey, Fadol, Sloane, and Villagomez are master's-prepared and are practicing in a variety of clinical facilities. Nichols has a BSN and was collaborating with others in this research project. These people appear to have research and clinical expertise to conduct this study.

3. Bruce is a master's-prepared (MSN) nurse who is providing care to people who have a history of hyperlipidemia and coronary artery disease. Grove is doctorally-prepared (PhD) in nursing and has co-authored two nursing research textbooks. These authors have strong educational preparation and sufficient clinical expertise to collaborate on a research project.

CHAPTER 2
INTRODUCTION TO THE QUANTITATIVE RESEARCH PROCESS

RELEVANT TERMS

1. n
2. s
3. b
4. e
5. r
6. d
7. k
8. q
9. h
10. l
11. m
12. c
13. t
14. a
15. o
16. p
17. j
18. i
19. g
20. f

KEY IDEAS

Control in Quantitative Research

1. highly controlled
2. quasi-experimental, experimental
3. descriptive, correlational
4. experimental
5. nonrandom, random
6. natural
7. highly controlled

8. experimental
9. partially controlled
10. quasi-experimental

Steps of the Research Process

1. problem-solving, nursing
2. problem, purpose
3. methodology
4. evaluation, revision, outcomes, communication of findings, and use of findings in practice
5. Step 1: research problem and purpose
   Step 2: literature review
   Step 3: study framework
   Step 4: research objectives, questions, or hypotheses
   Step 5: study variables
   Step 6: assumptions
   Step 7: limitations
   Step 8: research design
   Step 9: population and sample
   Step 10: methods of measurement
   Step 11: data collection
   Step 12: data analysis
   Step 13: research outcomes, communication of findings, and use of findings in practice
6. statements taken for granted or considered true, even though they have not been scientifically tested
7. You could identify any four of the following assumptions. (Williams, M. A. (1980) Editorial: Assumptions in research. *Research in Nursing & Health*, *3*(2), p. 48.)
   a. People want to assume control of their own health problems.
   b. Stress should be avoided.
   c. People are aware of the experiences that most affect their life choices.
   d. Health is a priority for most people.
   e. People in underserved areas feel underserved.
   f. Most measurable attitudes are held strongly enough to direct behavior.
   g. Health professionals view health care in a different manner than do lay persons.
   h. Human biological and chemical factors show less variation than do cultural and social factors.
   i. The nursing process is the best way of conceptualizing nursing practice.
   j. Statistically significant differences relate to the variable or variables under consideration.
   k. People operate on the basis of cognitive information.
   l. Increased knowledge about an event lowers anxiety about the event.
   m. Receipt of health care at home is preferable to receipt of care in an institution.
8. theoretical, methodological

9. Answer can include methodological or theoretical limitations. The methodological limitations include factors such as unrepresentative sample, small sample size, weak designs, single settings, instruments with limited reliability and validity, limited control over data collection, weak implementation of the treatment, and improper use of statistical analyses. Theoretical limitations include weak definitions of concepts in framework, weak conceptual definitions of variables, poorly developed study framework, or unclear link between study variables and framework concepts.

10. a smaller version of a proposed study conducted to develop and/or refine the methodology, such as the treatment, instruments, or data collection process to be used in the larger study

11. You could identify any five of the following reasons for conducting a pilot study.
    a. To determine whether the proposed study is feasible (*e.g,* Are the subjects available? Does the researcher have the time and money to do the study?).
    b. To develop or refine a research treatment.
    c. To develop a protocol for the implementation of a treatment.
    d. To identify problems with the design.
    e. To determine whether the sample is representative of the population or whether the sampling technique is effective.
    f. To examine the reliability and validity of the research instruments.
    g. To develop or refine data collection instruments.
    h. To refine the data collection and analysis plan.
    i. To give the researcher experience with the subjects, setting, methodology, and methods of measurement.
    j. To try out data analysis techniques.

Reading Research Reports

1. You could identify any three of the following research journals.
   a. *Advances in Nursing Science*
   b. *Applied Nursing Research*
   c. *Clinical Nursing Research: An International Journal*
   d. *Image: Journal of Nursing Scholarship*
   e. *Nursing Research*
   f. *Research in Nursing & Health*
   g. *Scholarly Inquiry for Nursing Practice: An International Journal*
   h. *Western Journal of Nursing Research*

2. You could identify any three of the following journals. A complete list of the journals in which research reports compose 50% or more of the journal content are in Table 2–3 of Chapter 2.
   a. *Issues in Comprehensive Pediatric Nursing*
   b. *Journal of Transcultural Nursing*
   c. *Heart & Lung: Journal of Critical Care*
   d. *Journal of Nursing Education*
   e. *Birth*
   f. *Nursing Diagnosis*

g. *Public Health Nursing*
h. *The Diabetes Educator*
i. *Maternal-Child Nursing Journal*
j. *Journal of Nursing Education*
3. introduction, methods, results, discussion
4. design, sample, setting, methods of measurement, data collection process
5. major findings, limitations of the study, conclusions drawn from the findings, implications of the findings for nursing, and recommendations for further research.
6. introduction section
7. theories, studies
8. skimming, comprehending, analyzing
9. comprehending
10. analyzing

MAKING CONNECTIONS

Types of Quantitative Research

1. c	11. b
2. a	12. a
3. b	13. c
4. a	14. a
5. c	15. c
6. d	16. a
7. a	17. b
8. b	18. a
9. c	19. a
10. d	20. b

PUZZLES

Word Scramble

1. Quantitative research methods include descriptive, correlational, quasi-experimental, and experimental studies.
2. Rigor and control are important in quantitative research.

Crossword Puzzle

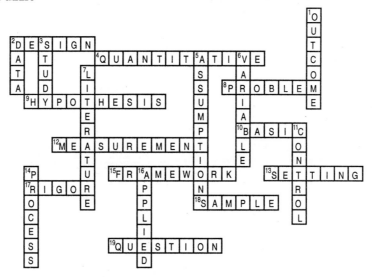

EXERCISES IN CRITIQUE

Type of Quantitative Research

1. c
2. c
3. a

Type of Setting

4. a
5. b
6. a

Type of Research Conducted

7. a
8. a
9. a

CHAPTER 3
RESEARCH PROBLEMS, PURPOSES,
AND HYPOTHESES

RELEVANT TERMS

Chapter Terms

1. f
2. i
3. h
4. g
5. k
6. j

7. e
8. d
9. a
10. c
11. b

Types of Hypotheses

1. h
2. g
3. b
4. e

5. c
6. a
7. d
8. f

Related to Variables

1. a
2. d
3. f

4. c
5. e
6. b

KEY IDEAS

Research Problem and Purpose

1. variables, population, setting
2. has an impact on nursing practice, builds on previous research, promotes theory development, addresses current concerns or priorities in nursing
3. You might identify any of the following agencies or organizations: National Institute for
   Nursing Research (NINR), American Association of Critical-Care Nurses (AACN),
   American Association of Occupational Health Nurses (AAOHN), Oncology Nursing
   Society (ONS), American Organization of Nurse Executives (AONE), or Agency for
   Health Care Policy and Research (AHCPR).
4. a. researchers' expertise
   b. money commitment
   c. availability of subjects, facility, and equipment
   d. study's ethical considerations

5. educational, clinical
6. research objectives, research questions, research hypotheses

EXERCISES IN CRITIQUE

Berg, *et al.,* Study

1. "Approximately 12 million Americans have asthma (National Center for Health Statistics, 1993). Asthma contributes substantially to morbidity and mortality. Indeed, according to National Health Statistics, the death rate attributable to asthma nearly doubled between 1979 and 1987 (National Center for Health, 1993). Strunk (1989) and other asthma specialists suggest that many of these deaths can be prevented by focusing on the behavioral factors which influence the self-management of asthma.

   One component of self-management is compliance with the medical regimen. Non-compliance has been shown to increase mortality and morbidity (Spector et al., 1986). The problem of managing compliance is complicated by the finding that patients over-estimate their own compliance with the recommended regimen. . . . Thus, interventions aimed at improving compliance need to address the issue of patients' recognition and/or reporting of their regimen behaviors" (pp. 225–226). ". . . More studies are needed to assess the impact of rural dwelling on those with asthma" (p. 227).
2. "The purpose of this study was to evaluate the impact of a nurse-administered asthma self-management program on patient compliance, asthma symptoms, and airway obstruction among patients treated in a rural setting" (p. 226).
3. The problem and purpose of the Berg, *et al.* (1997) study are significant. The problem and purpose provide the basis for the generation of hypotheses that are used to direct the study. This is a quasi-experimental study that will add to the knowledge base for the management of patients with asthma. This is an applied study, and the findings can have direct implications for nursing practice. The study is soundly based on previous research. This is a significant study because of the incidence of and the morbidity and mortality with asthma. Additional research is essential to improve patients' self-management of their chronic disease.
4. a. self-management program, patient compliance, asthma symptoms, and airway obstruction
   b. patients with asthma
   c. rural area
5. The study has a feasible purpose. The authors had access to an adequate sample, developed an ethical study, and identified appropriate measurement methods. The researchers had previously conducted studies in this area and had adequate educational preparation and clinical expertise. "This study was supported by NINR grant # 5–F3INR06787-02 and Glaxo Pharmaceutical grant #NUR005" (p. 225).

Lewis, *et al.,* Study

1. "Backrubs and changes in body position are established interventions for enhancing patients' comfort, mobilizing pulmonary secretions, and improving tissue perfusion through pressure reduction. Understanding the best strategies for combining these

interventions may improve patients' outcomes and make the best use of nursing time. Patients are commonly repositioned to the supine, right lateral, and left lateral positions before a backrub. The physiological effect of these interventions is questioned only if untoward changes are noted. Vital signs are routinely used to assess patients' responses to interventions such as changes in position and backrubs. Another useful measurement is mixed venous oxygen saturation (SvO_2), an indicator of oxygen delivery and consumption. Normally, patients are given a backrub immediately after a change in body position. The consequences of multiple, sequential activities can be hemodynamic compromise. We were interested in comparing the effects on SvO_2 of turning with immediate backrub and turning with a delayed backrub" (pp. 132–133). This problem is expressed in the first few paragraphs of the article.

2. The purpose of this study was "to examine the effect of a change in body position (right or left lateral) and timing of backrub (immediate or delayed) on mixed venous oxygen saturation in surgical ICU patients" (p. 132).

3. The problem and purpose are significant and provide a basis for the generation of research questions that guide the remaining steps of the study. The study focuses on nursing interventions (backrub and positioning) and produces significant findings that can be used in the care of ICU patients. The importance of this research is to determine how to maximize nursing interventions to optimize oxygenation and prevent an imbalance between oxygen supply and demand in the ICU patient.

4. a. body position (right or left lateral), timing of backrub (immediate or delayed), and mixed venous oxygen saturation
   b. surgical ICU patients
   c. ICU

5. The authors have strong educational preparation and clinical expertise and have conducted and published previous research in this area. The authors had access to an adequate, critically ill, male patient population at the Veterans Affairs Medical Center, Houston, Texas. The study was ethical and required limited equipment because the pulmonary artery catheters were already in place for the measurement of SvO_2. The treatments of positioning and backrub were within the practice realm of the nurse.

Bruce & Grove Study

1. "Cardiovascular diseases cause nearly one of every two deaths in adults 45 years and older . . . It ranks first in terms of social security disability and second only to all forms of arthritis for limitation of activity, and to all forms of cancer combined for total hospital stays. In direct health care costs, lost wages, and productivity, coronary artery disease (CAD) costs the United States more than $60 billion a year . . . Risk factors for CAD include male gender, family history of premature CAD, diabetes mellitus, hypertension, high cholesterol, cigarette smoking, and obesity . . . Education can promote changes in daily living that reduce the risk for CAD . . . The goal of all risk-factor reduction strategies is to change blood lipid profiles from a 'bad' one (high LDL, low HDL) to a 'good' one (low LDL, high HDL)" (Bruce & Grove, 1994, p. 67). This study problem was clearly stated in the first paragraph of the article.

2. "The purpose of this study was to compare a military population's mean levels of total serum cholesterol, LDL, HDL, and risk for cardiovascular disease (based on serum lipid levels) before and six months after a coronary artery risk evaluation (C.A.R.E.) program" (Bruce & Grove, 1994, p. 67).

3. The problem is significant to nursing because the C.A.R.E. program could be implemented by nurses in practice to improve the outcomes for patients with CAD. This could decrease the cost of health care and increase the patients' quality of life. This study builds on a solid base of previous research.

4. a. C.A.R.E. program, LDL, HDL, total serum cholesterol, and risk for cardiovascular disease
   b. military men and women
   c. outpatient primary care clinic of a 140-bed military hospital

5. The study was feasible because of the availability of a large number of subjects through the outpatient clinic. In addition, the military hospital provided the equipment and facility needed to conduct the study. The researchers demonstrated the educational preparation and clinical expertise to conduct this study. The study was conducted ethically with the protection of subjects' rights.

MAKING CONNECTIONS

Objectives, Questions, and Hypotheses

1. b, c, d, g
2. a, c, e, g
3. b, c, e, f
4. a, d, g, h
5. b, d, g, h
6. b, c, d, g
7. a, c, e, g
8. b, c, e, f
9. a, c, e, g
10. b, d, g, h
11. Low-back massage is no more effective in decreasing perceptions of low-back pain than no massage in patients with chronic low-back pain.
12. Increased age, decreased family support, and decreased health status are related to decreased self-care abilities of nursing home residents.
13. Nurses' perceived work stress, internal locus of control, and social support are not related to their psychological symptoms.

EXERCISES IN CRITIQUE

Berg *et al.,* Study

1. Hypotheses: "subjects receiving a self-management program would: increase compliance with inhaled medication, decrease the frequency of asthma symptoms, increase the percentage of symptoms-free days, and decrease airway obstruction. Secondary hypotheses were that subjects receiving the program would have increased self-efficacy and increased self-management behaviors" (p. 227).
2. Hypotheses clearly predict the outcomes for the study and provide direction for the remaining steps of the study. The variables identified in the purpose are also included in the hypotheses. The hypotheses are testable because they contain variables that can be manipulated and measured in the real world and can be supported or not supported based on the data collection and analysis. Stating hypotheses in the present tense does not limit them to the study being conducted and enables them to be used in additional research.

Lewis, *et al.,* Study

1. Research questions: "1. Does the change in SvO_2 after a 1-minute backrub in critically ill patients given the backrub immediately after turning differ from the change in SvO_2 in patients given the backrub 5 minutes after turning? 2. What is the effect of right and left lateral positions on SvO_2 in critically ill patients?" (p. 133)
2. The questions are clearly stated, reflective of the purpose, and provide direction for the conduct of the study. Since this is a quasi-experimental study, the authors might have provided clearer direction for their study with the statement of hypotheses versus research questions.

Bruce & Grove Study

1. Research question: "What is the difference in the mean total serum cholesterol, LDL cholesterol, and HDL cholesterol and cardiovascular risk levels of military members before and after participation in the C.A.R.E. program?" (Bruce and Grove, 1994, p. 68).
2. This question is clearly stated, includes the appropriate study variables, and directs the remaining steps of the research process.

MAKING CONNECTIONS

Understanding Study Variables

1. a
2. b
3. c
4. a
5. b
6. b
7. c
8. c
9. a
10. b
11. a
12. a

EXERCISES IN CRITIQUE

Berg, *et al.* Study

1. Independent variable: self-management program
   Dependent variables: compliance with inhaled medications, frequency of asthma symptoms, percentage of symptom-free days, airway obstruction, and self-efficacy and self-management behaviors.
2. Independent variable: self-management program
   Conceptual definition: "Self-management programs encourage the participation of the patient in the daily management of a chronic illness and are based on behavioral and social learning theory" (p. 226).
   Operational definition: "Self-management intervention. The self-management program was adapted from a program designed by Creer, Reynolds, and Kotses (1992) and consisted of 6 sessions, which included information about self-management behaviors and skills, asthma medications, asthma triggers, prevention of asthma attacks, relaxation techniques, psychological response to asthma, and problem-solving skills" (pp 228, 230).
   Dependent variable: compliance with inhaled medications
   Conceptual definition: Direct outcome to determine patients' management of their asthma with medication.
   Operational definition: "Metered Dose Inhaler (MDI) Chronolog is a monitoring device which is designed to house an MDI and used to assess compliance. Each time a subject uses the inhaler, a microswitch is activated and the Chronolog records the date and the time. Summary output data show the date and time of each subject activation for the period monitored . . . Compliance scores were calculated for each day and ranged from 0 to 100%" (pp. 230-231).
3. The conceptual and operational definitions of self-management program are clearly expressed in the article. The operational definition is based on the conceptual definition and can be manipulated in the study. The conceptual definition for compliance with inhaled medications is not clearly expressed and must be abstracted from the literature review. The operational definition of this variable is clearly expressed and is a precise measurement of compliance with inhaled medication.

Lewis, *et al.* Study

1. Independent variables: body position (right or left lateral) and timing of backrub (immediate or delayed)
   Dependent variable: mixed venous oxygen saturation (SvO_2)
2. Independent variable: body position
   Conceptual definition: "Nursing intervention to promote patients' comfort, mobilizing pulmonary secretions, and improving tissue perfusion through pressure reduction. . . . Routine nursing care such as turning the patient, suctioning, weighing, bed baths, and backrubs may cause increased oxygen consumption" (pp. 132, 133).
   Operational definition: intervention in which the "patient was turned to the left or right

lateral position. A single data collector turned the patient and placed two folded standard pillows, one pillow behind the patient's back and one between the patient's knees" (p. 135).
3. Conceptual definition is abstracted from the problem and the study framework. The operational definition is clearly expressed and controlled in implementation by one data collector who did all the patient body positioning.

Bruce & Grove Study

1. Independent variable: C.A.R.E. program
Dependent variables: total cholesterol, HDL, LDL, and cardiovascular risk level
2. C.A.R.E. program
Conceptual definition: Health screening and educational program designed to effect positive health outcomes (reduction in CAD risk) in people.
Operational definition: The C.A.R.E. program was implemented according to the guidelines in Figure 1 of the article (Bruce & Grove, 1994, p. 70).
3. The conceptual and operational definitions of the C.A.R.E. program are clearly presented in the article. All the dependent variables are clearly operationally defined, but the conceptual definitions might have been clearer.

CHAPTER 4
REVIEW OF LITERATURE

RELEVANT TERMS

1. m	10. c
2. j	11. l
3. o	12. q
4. p	13. r
5. e	14. h
6. k	15. g
7. n	16. a
8. d	17. b
9. i	18. f

KEY IDEAS

1. theoretical, empirical
2. compare and combine findings from the study with the literature to determine current knowledge of a phenomenon.
3. ethnographic and quantitative research (descriptive, correlational, quasi-experimental, and experimental studies)

4. historical research
5. landmark
6. replicated
7. approximate
8. secondary source
9. a. using the library
   b. identifying relevant sources
   c. locating research sources
   d. summarizing the research literature
10. academic libraries, special libraries
11. catalog listings, indexes, abstracts, and bibliographies
12. *Cumulative Index to Nursing & Allied Health Literature* (CINAHL)
13. Internet
14. *CINAHL Information System*, MEDLARS (*MEDical Literature Analysis and Retrieval System*), and MEDLINE (*MEDical Literature analysis and retrieval system onLINE*)
15. *Annual Review of Nursing Research*
16. synthesis
17. introduction, empirical literature, summary
18. core rewarming, cardiac surgery rewarming, radiant heat rewarming, forced air rewarming, rewarming after surgery, peripheral hypothermia, vasoconstriction, and postoperative period
19. urinary incontinence, daytime incontinence, nighttime incontinence, urinary incontinence management, prompted voiding, nursing home residents
20. a. organizing a list of sources
    b. searching the library for these sources
    c. systematically recording the references

MAKING CONNECTIONS

Theoretical and Empirical Sources

1. T		7. E
2. E		8. E
3. E		9. T
4. T		10. T
5. T		11. E
6. E		

Primary and Secondary Sources

1. S		6. P
2. P		7. P
3. P		8. S
4. S		9. P
5. S		10. P

EXERCISES IN CRITIQUE

1. a. name of the journal
   b. year the study was published
   c. volume number of the journal
   d. pages of the article
   e. issue number of the journal
   f. Bruce & Grove
   g. The effect of a coronary artery risk evaluation program on serum lipid values and cardiovascular risk levels
2. Berg, J., Dunbar-Jacob, J., & Sereika, S. M. (1997). An evaluation of a self-management program for adults with asthma. *Clinical Nursing Research, 6*(3), 225-238.
3. a. title and pages of the article
   b. volume number of the journal and pages of the article
   c. year the article was published and volume and issue numbers of the journal
4. a. No separate section. Review of literature is part of the introduction of the article.
   b. Literature Review
   c. Background
5. Yes, relevant studies are identified and described. According to the introduction section and the references of the Berg, *et al.,* (1997) study, it appears that they identified and described at least 6 relevant studies in their literature review. The studies cited as part of their literature review include: Spector, *et al.,* 1986; Glanz, Stanley, Swartz, & Francis, 1984; Lorig & Holman, 1989; Creer, 1991; Wing, Epstein, Nowalk, & Lamparski, 1986; O'Leary, Shoor, Lorig, & Holman, 1988.
6. Berg, *et al.,* (1997) examined the proposition that perceived self-efficacy expectancies have a strong influence on chronically ill patients' ability to manage their own care. Two theoretical sources cited in the literature review are Holroyd & Creer, 1986; O'Leary, 1985.
7. primary source
8. Dunbar, J. (1980). Adhering to medical advice: A review. *International Journal of Mental Health*, 9, 70–87.
9. The sources are fairly current, but no sources from 1994–1997 were cited. The references range from 1959 through 1993. The article was published late in 1997 and there is no indication of when the study was originally submitted or accepted for publication. A review of the literature after the conduct of the study might have identified some more current sources from 1994–1997. The sources cited seem relevant to the topic, and 11 of the 26 sources, or 42%, were published in 1990s.
10. The Berg, *et al.* (1997) study does not have a separate review of literature section; the literature is summarized in the introduction section of the article. Several relevant studies are cited, but no sources from 1994–1996 were identified. There is limited coverage of what is not known about the self-management program for adults with asthma. Thus, the literature review for this study might have been expanded to provide the reader with a clearer understanding of how this study will add to nursing's current knowledge base.

11. Yes, relevant studies are identified and described. The Lewis, *et al.,* (1997) Literature Review Section and References cite at least 10 studies. Some of the research sources include Shively, 1988; Tidwell, Ryan, Osguthorpe, Paull, & Smith, 1990; Winslow, Clark, White, & Tyler, 1990; Copel & Stolarik, 1991; Atkins, Hapshe, & Riegel, 1994; Tyler, Winslow, Clark, & White, 1990.

12. Lewis, *et al.* (1997) indicated that the framework for their study was based on the physiological principles of underlying SvO_2. They cited three theoretical sources that were physiologically focused in their Framework Section: Ahrens & Rutherford, 1993; Cernaianu & Nelson, 1993; White, Winslow, Clark, & Tyler, 1990

13. secondary source, primary source

14. The Lewis, *et al.* (1997) study has current sources. The references ranged from 1982 through 1994, and the article was published in early 1997. There is no indication of when the article was submitted or accepted for publication, which might account for the last reference being in 1994. Nine of the 15 sources, or 60%, were published in the 1990s, and four of these were published in 1993–1994.

15. Lewis, *et al.,* (1997) provide detailed coverage of relevant studies (pp. 133–134) and also a clear summary of what is known. "In summary, nursing interventions cause a significant decrease in SvO_2 immediately after the intervention is started. SvO_2 values usually return to baseline within 3 to 9 minutes, depending on the intervention" (p. 134). However, their review of literature would have been stronger if they had indicated what is not known and how their study will contribute to the development of nursing knowledge in the area studied.

16. By examining the background section and the references of the Bruce & Grove article, you will note that they identified and described 15 studies. Some of those studies were by Blair, Bryant, & Bocuzzi (1988); Blankenhorn, Nessim, Johnson, San Marco, Azen, & Cashen-Hemphill (1987); Bruno, Arnold, Winick, & Wynder (1983); Freidewald, Levy, & Fredrickson (1972); Lipid Research Clinics Program (1984).

17. Bruce & Grove (1994) cited physiological, pathological, and health education theoretical sources to support their study. Some of the theoretical sources include American Heart Association (1988); Green Kreuter, Deeds, & Partiridge (1980); Kwiterovick (1989). *Note from author:* Some of the theoretical content and sources were deleted at the request of the journal editor to shorten the article and increase the appeal to the journal audience.

18. secondary source, primary source

19. The references range from 1947 through 1990. The article was published in 1994, so the authors' sources are at least four years old. However, this article was submitted in 1992, accepted for publication in 1993, and published in 1994. The delay between submitting the article and publication can make some of the references less current. More than 50% of the sources were from the late 1980s.

20. Bruce & Grove clearly summarize what is known and not known about the effects of educational programs on adults' serum lipid values and cardiovascular risk levels. The study by Blair, Bryant, & Bocuzzi (1988) highlights the effectiveness of nursing intervention in individuals with hyperlipidemia. The authors indicate how their study will add to the current knowledge base is this area of study.

—————————:••●●••:—————————

CHAPTER 5
UNDERSTANDING THEORY AND
RESEARCH FRAMEWORKS

RELEVANT TERMS

Check the glossary in the back of your text for definitions.

KEY IDEAS

1. organize what we know about a phenomenon
2. determining the truth of each relational statement in the theory
3. conceptual models
4. theory
5. disconnected
6. the framework
7. concepts
8. constructs
9. variable
10. propositions
11. hypotheses
12. explain which concepts contribute to or partially cause an outcome
13. all of the major concepts in a theory or framework linked together by arrows expressing the proposed linkages between the concepts
14. research tradition

MAKING CONNECTIONS

1. e	4. h	7. i
2. b	5. c	8. g
3. a	6. d	9. f

PUZZLES

Word Scramble

Many studies are required to validate all of the statements in a theory.

Secret Message

You need to determine links among the conceptual definitions, the variables in the study, and the related measurement methods.

Crossword Puzzle

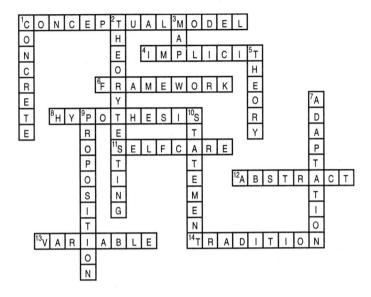

EXERCISES IN CRITIQUE

1. SvO_2, oxygen supply, tissue oxygen demands, SaO_2, hemoglobin level, cardiac output, tissue oxygen consumption, routine nursing care, patient conditions

2. SvO_2—mixed venous oxygen saturation
   oxygen supply—not defined
   tissue oxygen demand—not defined
   SaO_2—arterial oxygen saturation
   hemoglobin level—not defined
   cardiac output—not defined
   tissue oxygen consumption—not defined
   routine nursing care—not defined
   patient conditions—not defined

3.

CONCEPT	VARIABLE	MEASUREMENT
SvO_2	SvO_2	fiber-optic theromdilution pulmonary artery catheter measures
oxygen supply		
tissue oxygen demand		
SaO_2		
hemoglobin level		
cardiac output		
tissue oxygen consumption		
routine nursing care	position of patient	turning patient to right or left
immediacy of backrub	immediate or delayed backrub	
patient conditions		

4. Measurement methods are consistent with concepts. However, conceptual definitions are not provided and cannot be compared.
5. An uncompensated reduction in SaO_2, hemoglobin level, or cardiac output or increases in tissue oxygen consumption will result in a decreased SvO_2.

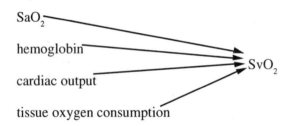

$$SaO_2$$
$$hemoglobin$$
$$cardiac\ output$$
$$tissue\ oxygen\ consumption$$
$$\rightarrow SvO_2$$

The SaO_2 influences the SvO_2.

$$SaO_2 \longrightarrow SvO_2$$

Pathological pulmonary conditions that impair oxygen transfer at the alveolar-capillary membrane will result in less oxygen available for transport through the circulation.

$$patient\ condition \longrightarrow oxygen\ supply$$

A deficit in hemoglobin reduces the oxygen-binding capacity of the blood and affects oxygen supply to the tissues.

$$hemoglobin \longrightarrow oxygen\ supply$$

Cardiac output is the means for transporting oxyhemoglobin through the system.

cardiac output ⟶ oxygen supply

Tissue extraction of oxygen is increased in conditions such as fever, seizures, and shivering.

patient condition ⟶ tissue oxygen consumption

Routine nursing care such as turning the patient, suctioning, weighing, bed baths, and backrubs may cause increased oxygen consumption.

routine nursing care ⟶ tissue oxygen consumption

6. Proposition: Routine nursing care such as turning the patient, suctioning, weighing, bed baths, and backrubs may cause increased oxygen consumption.

   Research Question: Does the change in SvO_2 after a 1-minute backrub in critically ill patients given the backrub immediately after turning differ from the change in SvO_2 in patients given the backrub 5 minutes after turning?

   Research Question: What is the effect of right and left lateral positions in SvO_2 in critically ill patients?

7. The proposition is tested by the study design by testing differences in the effect of providing backrubs immediately after turning and 5 minutes after turning, and by testing differences in the effect of turning the patient to the right and to the left.

8. The framework is not expressed as a conceptual map. A possible map of the framework is shown below:

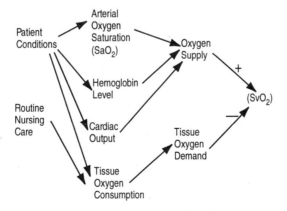

9. References from the literature: Effects of nursing care on oxygen consumption
    Shively (1998)
    Tidwell, Ryan, Psguthorpe, Paull, & Smith (1990)
    Winslow, Clark, & White (1990)
    Copel & Stolarik (1991)
    Atkins, Hapshe, & Riegel (1994)
    Tyler, Winslow, Clark, & White (1990)
    No other relationships are validated from the literature.
10. Paragraphs will vary but should include the following points:
    The framework expresses the causal linkages associated with SvO_2. Conceptual definitions are not provided. This commonly occurs with physiologic concepts because the concepts are assumed by the author to have a common meaning that will be known by the readers. Relationships between concepts are not presented in theoretical form and are somewhat difficult to sort out from the discussion provided. No conceptual map is provided.

CHAPTER 6
EXAMINING ETHICS IN NURSING RESEARCH

RELEVANT TERMS

1. f
2. a
3. g
4. i
5. h
6. d
7. j
8. b
9. l
10. e
11. c
12. k

KEY IDEAS

1. a. disclosure of essential study information to the subject
    b. comprehension of this information by the subject
    c. competency of the subject to give consent
    d. voluntary consent by the subject to participate in the study

2. You might have identified any of the following:
   - introduction of the research activities
   - statement of the research purpose
   - explanation of study procedures
   - description of risks and discomforts
   - description of benefits
   - disclosure of alternatives
   - assurance of anonymity and confidentiality
   - offer to answer questions
   - option to withdraw
3. voluntary
4. incompetent
5. institutional review board (IRB)
6. a. exempt from review
   b. expedited review
   c. complete or full review
7. To determine the benefit-risk ratio, you need to assess the benefits and risks of the sampling method, consent process, procedures, and outcomes of the study. Informed consent must be obtained from the subjects, and selection and treatment of the subjects during the study must be fair. The type of knowledge generated from the study also needs to be examined to determine how this knowledge will impact the subject and influence nursing practice. The risks need to be reduced if possible and should not cause serious harm to the subjects; the benefits need to be maximized. Then the risks and benefits are examined; the benefits need to out weigh the risks adequately for the study to be considered ethical to conduct.
8. exempt from review or expedited review
9. complete review
10. Any three of the following could be identified: fabrication, falsification, or forging of data; manipulation of the design or methods; selective retaining or manipulating data; or plagiarism.
11. Office of Scientific Integrity Review (OSIR) and Office of Scientific Integrity (OSI)
12. Yes. This is an area of concern in nursing, and articles have been published outlining the concerns and actions to be taken to control scientific misconduct. None of the major misconduct problems mentioned in the text has been in nursing.
13. Yes. An increasing number of animals are being used by nurse scientists to generate basic research knowledge for the profession.
14. American Association for Accreditation of Laboratory Animal Care (AAALAC)
15. If your answer is yes, your rationale might focus on the importance of animal studies to generate basic knowledge and the fact that these studies provide the basis for conducting applied studies on humans. Agencies exist to protect the animals and ensure humane treatment during research.
    If your answer is no, your rationale might focus on the inhuman aspects of using animals as research subjects.

MAKING CONNECTIONS

Historical Events, Ethical Codes, and Regulation

1. b
2. c
3. d
4. b
5. c

6. a
7. d
8. b
9. a
10. c

PUZZLES

Crossword Puzzle

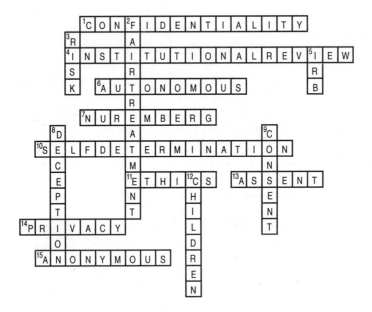

EXERCISES IN CRITIQUE

1. The Berg, *et al.* (1997) study indicates that informed consent was obtained from each subject but does not indicate how this was accomplished. In addition, there is no indication that the study was reviewed by an Institutional Review Board (IRB). This study appears to be ethical when examining the benefit-risk ratio, but the authors might have provided more information about the approval process for conducting this study.

2. Lewis, *et al.,* (1997) identified the following process for identifying their subjects and obtaining their consent to participate in their study: "Brochures were placed in physician offices and pharmacies, and information about the study was announced on the radio and in newspapers. Potential subjects were called after they indicated an interest in participation. Of 136 adults screened, 87 (64%) were eligible for inclusion. Sixty-eight (78%) signed consent forms were returned" (Lewis, *et al.,* 1997, p. 228). The authors do not indicate how they obtained permission to advertise their studies in the different locations. They need to discuss their approval by an Institutional Review Board if appropriate. This study appears to be ethical, since the risks are minimal and the benefits are strong and the authors indicated that signed consent forms were obtained from the subjects. However, the ethical review process might have been discussed in more depth.

3. Bruce & Grove indicated that the "Strategic Air Command Surgeon General mandated the educational program (institutional review) be provided to the military members and dependents and participation in the study was voluntary" (Bruce & Grove, 1994, p. 69). The study was ethical because the researchers obtained institutional approval and signed consent from the subjects who voluntarily participated in the study. In addition, the risks were minimal and the benefits were strong in this study.

CHAPTER 7
CLARIFYING RESEARCH DESIGNS

RELEVANT TERMS

Check the glossary in the back of your text for definitions.

KEY IDEAS

1. effects
2. cause, effect, cause
3. biases
4. control
5. treatment
6. threats to validity
7. cause and effect
8. comparisons
9. comparisons

MAKING CONNECTIONS

Matching Definitions

1. g	4. a	7. d
2. h	5. f	8. b
3. i	6. c	9. e

Matching Designs

1. a	5. b	8. h
2. c	6. i	9. g
3. f	7. e	10. d
4. f		

Mapping the Design

Design #1

Home Care For Terminal Cancer Patients

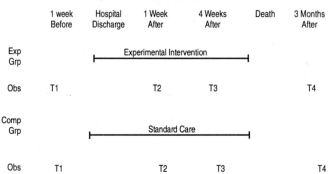

Design #2

Communication with Families in an ICU

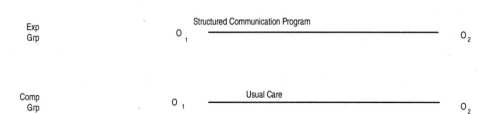

Design #3

Multidisciplinary Care Delivery

	1 Year	6 Months	6 Months

Retrospective
Chart
Review

NOM

Prospective
Study

OM   NOM   OM   NOM   OM   NOM

Propsective
Study

OM

OM = outcomes-managed approach
NOM = non-outcomes-managed approach

PUZZLES

Word Scramble

Just as a blueprint for a house must be individualized to the specific house being built, so must the design be made specific to a study.

Secret Message

The purpose of a design is to set up a situation that maximizes the possibilities of obtaining accurate answers to objectives, questions, or hypotheses.

Crossword Puzzle

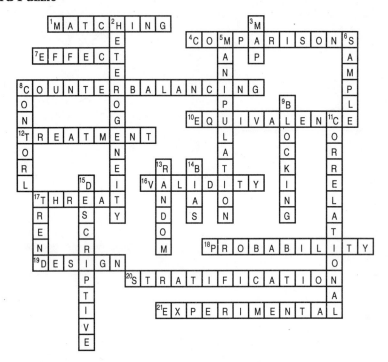

EXERCISES IN CRITIQUE

1. a. According to the criteria in this text, this is a quasi-experimental study; the authors refer to it as experimental.
   b. According to the criteria in this text, this is a quasi-experimental study; the authors refer to it as experimental.
   c. comparative descriptive
2. Sources of bias
   a. Berg, *et al.* study
   - Sample was not randomly selected. Although subjects were randomly assigned, convenience sampling was used. Subjects who volunteered may have been different from those who did not volunteer. For example, those who volunteered may have been more invested in self-management of their asthma than those who did not express interest in the study. The author does not address whether the sample is representative of people who have asthma.
   - Prior to initiation of the program, 19% of the sample withdrew because of weather problems or illness. It is possible that those who withdrew were different in important ways from those who remained in the study. For example, those who withdrew may have tended to be less compliant with treatment regimens.

- Measurement: the authors indicated a possible problem with measurement sensitivity.
- Subjects in the study were relatively well educated, which is important to note since the study uses an educational intervention.
- The authors suggest that the short duration of follow-up may not have been sufficient to detect changes.

  b. Lewis & colleagues' study
- Sample was not randomly selected. Subjects who volunteered may have been different from those who did not volunteer.
- The sample included only males, a consequence of conducting the study at a Veteran's Administration hospital.
- Other than gender, the author does not address whether the sample is representative of people being cared for in a surgical ICU.

  c. Bruce and Grove's study
- Sample was not randomly selected. Subjects who volunteered may have been different from those who did not volunteer.
- Ethnicity of the sample is not reported; thus the possibility of bias cannot be judged. The effectiveness of risk reduction strategies may differ in some ethnic groups due to genetic variation.
- Military personnel may differ from the general population in the likelihood that they will follow a risk reduction program.

3. a. You could have listed any three of the following:
- Controlling extraneous variables—subjects were excluded if they had other respiratory disorders or were current smokers.
- Subjects were classified according to asthma severity. A stratified random permuted block scheme was used to generate treatment assignments to allow equal distribution of asthma severity to the two groups.
- Treatment—the intervention had been used in previous studies and was scripted so that the treatment would be the same in the five groups conducted in the study.
- Controlling measurement—instruments with documented validity and reliability were used for measurement.

  b. You could have listed any three of the following:
- Controlling measurement—valid and reliable instruments were used. Physiologic measures were carefully controlled for consistency.
- Controlling extraneous variables—potential subjects were excluded if they were less than 18 years of age; had sepsis; had had a pneumonectomy, lobectomy or organ transplantation; had mechanical assist devices in place; or were using neuromuscular blocking agents.
- A nested design was used to examine interactions of turning and backrub.
- Intervention—the procedures for turning and backrub were carefully defined.
- A single data collector provided the intervention and collected the data for a patient.

  c. You could have listed any three of the following:
- Controlling the environment - subjects received a carefully designed treatment at one military base.

- Controlling equivalence—subjects were limited to those with serum cholesterol levels between 200 mg/dl and 300 mg/dl.
- Controlling treatment—a defined protocol was used as the treatment
- Controlling measurement—a standardized protocol for lipid data collection was followed by each subject.
- Subjects were excluded if they were diabetic or were being pharmacologically treated for hyperlipidemia.

4. a. Berg & colleagues' study
- Comparison of pretest compliance of subjects who received the experimental treatment and those who did not
- Comparison of posttest compliance of those who received the experimental treatment and those who did not
- Comparison of asthma severity between the two age groups
- Comparison of baseline average total daily symptoms
- Comparison of posttreatment average total daily symptoms
- Comparison of baseline percentage of symptom-free days
- Comparison of posttreatment percentage of symptom-free days
- Comparison of peak-flow measurements between the two groups
- Comparison of self-efficacy between the two groups
- Comparison of self-management between the two groups
- Comparison of self-reported compliance with compliance measured by the chronolog

   b. Lewis & colleagues' study
- Comparisons across timed measurements for each subject
- Comparisons of baseline values between the two groups
- Comparisons of left turns and right turns between the two groups, and for the total sample
- Comparisons of timing of backrub between the two groups and for the total sample
- Comparisons of the effect of turns and the effect of backrub for the total sample

   c. Bruce & Grove's study
- Risk levels of subjects before and after treatment using a standard protocol
- Comparison of cardiovascular risk and total cholesterol level
- Comparison of cardiovascular risk and LDL cholesterol
- Comparison of cardiovascular risk and HDL cholesterol

5. a. Berg & colleagues' study
- well-educated adult rural residents with asthma
- people receiving the same educational program used in the study

   b. Lewis & colleagues' study
- male patients being cared for in a surgical ICU who are similar to subjects in the study
- ICU patients receiving a backrub using the same procedure as that used in the study
- ICU patients being turned using the same procedure as that used in the study
- ICU patients with SvO_2 values similar to those of subjects in the study

- ICU patients with hemoglobin levels similar to those of subjects in the study
- ICU patients with hemodynamically stable conditions

c. Bruce & Grove's study: cardiovascular high risk patients

6. a. Berg & colleagues' study
   - possible lack of measurement sensitivity
   - the short duration of follow-up
   - convenience sample
   - interaction of selection and treatment, because of high educational level of subjects and high study mortality rate

   b. Lewis & colleagues' study: Interaction of selection and treatment: only patients who were hemodynamically stable were included in the study. The treatment may not have the same effect on patients who are unstable.

   c. Bruce & Grove's study: interaction of selection and treatment, because compliance of military personnel to treatment may be higher than that of general public

7. a. Berg & colleagues' study
   - randomized assignment to groups
   - stratification of subjects based on asthma severity
   - controlled treatment

   b. Lewis & colleagues' study
   - random assignment of subjects to groups
   - repeated measures
   - controlled treatment

   c. Bruce & Grove's study
   - carefully designed protocol
   - large sample size
   - control of measurement

CHAPTER 8
POPULATIONS AND SAMPLES

RELEVANT TERMS

1. j	8. i
2. a	9. l
3. n	10. b
4. g	11. d
5. k	12. e
6. f	13. h
7. m	14. c

KEY IDEAS

1. elements
2. target population
3. sample, accessible population, target population
4. You could have identified any two of the following.
   - compare the demographic characteristics of the sample with those of the target population
   - compare mean sample values of study variables with the values of the target population determined from previous research
   - determine sample mortality
   - evaluate the possibilities of systematic bias in the sample in terms of the setting, characteristics of the sample, and ranges of values on measured variables
5. the expected difference in values that occurs when different subjects from the same sample are examined
6. sampling frame
7. strategies used to obtain a sample for a study
8. You might choose any three of the following.
   - Did the researcher successfully implement the sampling plan?
   - Was the sampling plan effective in achieving representativeness?
   - Were the subjects selected from a sampling frame?
   - Were the subjects randomly selected?
   - If control and treatment groups were used, how were these groups selected?
9. homogeneous
10. heterogenous
11. sample criteria
12. sample characteristics
13. sample mortality
14. random
15. nonrandom
16. a. simple random sampling
    b. stratified random sampling
    c. cluster sampling
    d. systematic sampling
17. probability, nonprobability, probability
18. a. convenience sampling
    b. quota sampling
    c. purposive sampling
    d. network sampling
19. nonprobability
20. accidental sampling
21. judgmental sampling
22. power analysis
23. differences, relationships

24. .8
25. power analysis
26. null hypothesis
27. a. effect size of a study
    b. type of study
    c. number of variables
    d. measurement sensitivity
    e. data analysis techniques

MAKING CONNECTIONS

1. g
2. b and f
3. c
4. a
5. b
6. h
7. i
8. b

9. e
10. d
11. g
12. c
13. d
14. b
15. f and g

PUZZLES

Crossword Puzzle

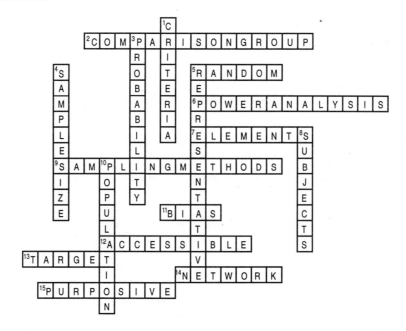

EXERCISES IN CRITIQUE

Bruce & Grove Study

1. "(a) greater than 16 years; (b) military members (active duty, retired, or dependent); (c) not under pharmacological treatment for hyperlipidemia; (d) English-speaking; (e) triglycerides under 400 mg/dl . . . ; (f) nondiabetic; and (g) no current referrals to other health providers" (Bruce & Grove, 1994, p. 69).

2. "The sample consisted of 92 men and 103 women and included 36 married couples. The subjects ranged from 20 to 80 years of age, with a mean age of 53.33 years (± 13 SD). Information about the subjects' body mass index (BMI), systolic blood pressure (SBP), diastolic blood pressure (DBP), heart rate, and glucose are provided in Table 1. Means for these variables were within normal limits" (Bruce & Grove, 1994, p. 69).

3. 195 subjects
   "Power analysis was performed to confirm the adequacy of the sample size" (Bruce and Grove, 1994, p. 69). However, the specifics of this analysis were deleted from the article at the request of the journal editor.

4. The sample size was adequate to examine four variables in this quasi-experimental study. Power analysis indicated that the sample size was adequate to detect differences. Very sensitive measurements were obtained of the total cholesterol, HDL, and LDL.

5. There was no sample mortality. A total of 483 subjects were screened, but only 195 became subjects and completed the study.

6. nonprobability

7. convenience sampling

8. The fact that the sample is not random potentially decreases its representativeness of the population. However, actively recruiting subjects and including all subjects that met the sample criteria increases the representativeness of this sample. The large sample size increases the representativeness of the sample.

9. Since the sample is nonrandom, the findings should be generalized to the accessible population and not the target population. However, these findings are extremely consistent with the extensive number of studies in this area, which increases the generalizability of the findings.

Berg, Dunbar-Jacob, & Sereika Study

1. "rural dwelling adults age 18 years and older with a medical diagnosis of asthma who were being treated with prescribed, regularly administered, inhaled medications other than as-needed bronchodilators" (p. 227).

2. "The subjects were predominantly female, Caucasian, and married . . . The subjects in the sample were relatively well educated. There were no significant differences found between groups on these characteristics" (p. 228). Subject characteristics are detailed in Table 1 of the article, which can be found in Appendix A.

3. 55 subjects
   "No previous intervention studies using similar compliance outcome measures reported the appropriate summary statistics of their data to estimate sample size. In light of this, approximations were made according to recommendations using Cohen (1998). The

significance level was set at .05 and the power level was set at .80. A moderate effect size of .5 was chosen, given the nature of the data and lack of pilot data" (p. 228).

4. The sample size does not appear to be adequate. There is a possibility of Type II errors in the study. Several of the study hypotheses were not supported. The authors suggest a possible problem with measurement sensitivity. Crude measures require larger sample sizes. A larger sample would have allowed testing for a smaller effect size, although the authors indicate that "the degree of improvement in adherence was not sufficient to produce a clinical impact" (p. 235).

5. Sixty-eight subjects signed consent forms. "Before the initiation of the program, 13 (19%) withdrew from the study due to weather problems and illness. . . Fifty-four subjects completed the program and 1 subject withdrew but was included in the analysis" (p. 228).

6. nonprobability

7. convenience sampling

8. The sample was not random, which decreases its probability of being representative of the population. The authors indicate that subjects had a relatively high level of education and were predominantly female, Caucasian, and married. Therefore, the sample does not appear to be representative.

9. The study used a nonrandom sample that does not appear to be representative, so the findings should be generalized only to the accessible population, not the target population.

Lewis & Colleagues Study

1. "Subjects who had a fiber-optic pulmonary artery catheter in place, a baseline SvO_2 of 50% or higher, and an indwelling arterial catheter with normal waveform were eligible for inclusion in the study. Exclusion criteria included age less than 18 years, sepsis, pneumonectomy or lobectomy, mechanical assist devices in place, organ transplantation, and use of neuromuscular blocking agents. No subjects were excluded because of advanced age" (p. 135).

2. The mean age of the subjects was 60.9 years (standard deviation [SD] = 8.6; range, 40–79 years). Forty-nine subjects had had aortocoronary bypass surgery; 6, resection of an aortic aneurysm; 1, atrial septal repair; and 1, an esophogastrectomy. All subjects were in the surgical ICU at the time of the intervention. Forty-nine subjects were receiving oxygen by either face mask ($n = 22$) or nasal cannula ($n = 27$). Four subjects were receiving mechanical ventilation; 3 of these were receiving 5 cm of positive end-expiratory pressure. The remaining 4 subjects had no supplemental oxygen therapy. Mean SaO_2, hemoglobin, cardiac output, and cardiac index are given in Table 1" (p. 136) (provided in the article in Appendix A).

3. 57 subjects.
"Power analysis for repeated measures indicates that 23 subjects are needed to detect a medium effect at the .05 level of significance with a power of 0.80 and an estimated mean correlation among the repeated measures of 0.50 when only seven repeated measures are collected. This study had two grouping variables: position and immediacy of backrub. A minimum of 23 subjects was recruited into each group. This sample size provided more than adequate power, because 15 repeated measures were recorded for each subject" (p. 134–135).

4. The study hypotheses were supported, and the sample size was adequate.
5. No sample mortality is reported.
6. nonprobability
7. convenience sampling
8. The sample was not random, which decreases its representativeness of the population studied. Women were not included in the sample, which decreases the sample's representativeness. The authors point out that only hemodynamically stable patients were included in the sample.
9. Since the sample is nonrandom, the findings need to be generalized to the accessible population. However, these findings were consistent with the findings of other studies, which increases the generalizability of the findings. The findings cannot be generalized to women or to patients who are hemodynamically unstable.

CHAPTER 9
MEASUREMENT AND DATA COLLECTION IN RESEARCH

RELEVANT TERMS
Check the glossary in the back of your text for definitions.

KEY IDEAS
1. trustworthy
2. true
3. error
4. direct
5. indirect
6. .80

Random Error
1. variations in administration of the measurement procedure
2. subjects completing a paper and pencil scale accidentally marking the wrong column
3. punching the wrong key while entering data into the computer

Systematic Error

1. a weight scale that weighs higher than it should
2. a thermometer that is not calibrated
3. failure to count two exam questions in calculating exam grades

Data Collection Tasks

1. selecting subjects
2. collecting data in a consistent way
3. maintaining research controls indicated by the study design
4. protecting the study integrity (or validity)
5. solving problems that threaten to disrupt the study

MAKING CONNECTIONS

Measurement Error

1. b
2. b
3. a
4. b
5. a

Type of Reliability or Validity

1. g
2. d
3. k
4. m
5. e
6. a
7. h
8. c
9. i
10. j
11. f
12. l
13. b

PUZZLES

Word Scramble

There is no perfect measure.

Secret Message

Reliability testing should be performed on each instrument used in a study.

Crossword Puzzle

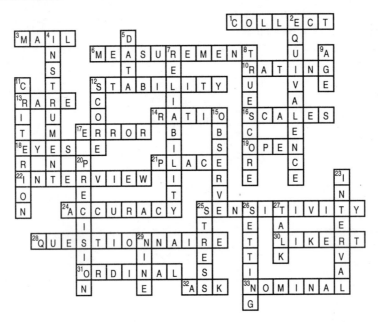

EXERCISES IN CRITIQUE

1. *For Berg, Dunbar-Jacob, & Sereika's study*

Variable	Method of Measurement	Directness
Compliance	MDI Chronolog	D
Compliance	journal of daily asthma concerns	I
Peak-flow	spirometrics peak-flow meter	D
Self-efficacy	the Self-Efficacy for Asthma Management Scale	I
Self-management	the Asthma Self-Management Assessment Tool	I

For Lewis & colleagues' study

Variable	Method of Measurement	Directness
SvO_2	fiber-optic thermodilution pulmonary artery catheter (the Explorer continuous venous oximeter, American Edwards Laboratories, Irvine, Calif)	D

For Bruce & Grove's study

Variable	Method of Measurement	Directness
total serum cholesterol	blood sample	D
LDL	blood sample	D
HDL	blood sample	D
risk level	calculated from other measures	D

2. *Berg, Dunbar-Jacob, & Sereika*
   a. Measure: MDI Chronolog.
      Developer: Forefront Engineering Corporation, Denver, CO
      Date developed: not provided
      Description of method of measurement: detailed and clear description of measurement
      Range of values: not provided
      Critique: Excellent description; reader has clear understanding of the process of measurement.
   b. Measure: Journal of Daily Asthma Concerns
      Developer: Creer
      Date developed: 1992
      Description of method of measurement: Diary: "Subjects were asked to complete information about medication-taking behavior on a daily basis. For the assessment of asthma symptoms, subjects were required to record information about the presence or absence of four different symptoms: sneeze, cough, shortness of breath, and chest tightness. Subjects also recorded information about the frequency of asthma attacks during daytime and nighttime, and peak-flow readings" (p. 231).
   c. Measure: Spirometrics Peak-Flow Meter
      Developer: Spirometric, Inc., Auburn, ME
      Date developed: not given
      Range of measures: 90–700 lpm
      Description of method of measurement: not provided

Critique: The authors assume that the reader is familiar with the use of peak-flow meters. The description of measurement is not adequate.

   d. Measure: The Self-Efficacy for Asthma Management Scale

   Developer: Developed by the authors for this study

   Date developed: not given

   Range of measures: 0–100

   Description of method of measurement: 14-item scale. No information provided on method of scaling or scoring the instrument.

   Critique: The description of measurement is not adequate.

   e. Measure: The Asthma Self-Management Assessment Tool

   Developer: Taylor and colleagues, modified by authors for present study

   Date developed: original tool published in 1991

   Range of measures: 0–33

   Description of method of measurement: "the tool contained scenarios for exercise-induced asthma, respiratory tract infections, and a severe asthma attack. Subjects identified their management strategies for each of three types of asthma episodes and were awarded points on the basis of critical incidents and levels of self-management" (p. 232).

   Critique: Information is not complete. However, details of points awarded probably would have required more space than that allowed by the editors.

Lewis & colleagues' study

   a. Measure: SvO_2 (the Explorer continuous venous oximeter)

   Developer: American Edwards laboratories, Irvine, California

   Date developed: not given

   Description of method of measurement: no description is provided.

   Critique: The authors assume that this measure is common knowledge. It is not clear from the presentation if a single value is obtained or if calculations are made from several measures that are obtained. No explanation is given of the functions of computers in calculating, storing, or displaying the measures.

Bruce & Grove's study

   a. Total Serum Cholesterol

   The Total Serum Cholesterol value was obtained from the patient's record. No information is provided on the equipment or method used to obtain the value. Since all the patients received care in the same setting, one could expect the procedure and equipment to be consistent across patients and thus, that values across patients were comparable. However, this is an assumption and is not documented. The authors do report that the National Bureau of Standards and the Centers for Disease Control establish standards that must be followed by laboratories in the measurement and reporting of laboratory values.

b. LDL

The LDL value was obtained from the patient's record. No information is provided on the equipment or method used to obtain the value. Since all the patients received care in the same setting, one could expect the procedure and equipment to be consistent across patients and thus, that values across patients were comparable. However, this is an assumption and is not documented. The authors do report that the National Bureau of Standards and the Centers for Disease Control establish standards that must be followed by laboratories in the measurement and reporting of laboratory values. The level of LDL was calculated using the following equation: Total Cholesterol – [HDL cholesterol + triglycerides/5] = LDL.

c. HDL

The HDL value was obtained from the patient's record. No information is provided on the equipment or method used to obtain the value. Since all the patients received care in the same setting, one could expect the procedure and equipment to be consistent across patients and thus, that values across patients were comparable. However, this is an assumption and is not documented. The authors do report that the National Bureau of Standards and the Centers for Disease Control establish standards that must be followed by laboratories in the measurement and reporting of laboratory values.

d. Estimated Cardiovascular Risk Level

The determination of cardiovascular risk level is not discussed in the measurement section of the paper. In the Procedure section, the authors state that each subject was determined to have low, moderate, or high risk for cardiovascular disease. The assessment of cardiac risk was performed by the program nurse in conjunction with the clinic physician, and was based on reported risk factors and the results of the serum lipid profile, according to the National Cholesterol Education Program (NCEP) guidelines. The nonlipid risk factors are not defined; however, the description of the sample lists "other reported risk factors" of cigarette smoking, hypertension, obesity, and diagnosed coronary artery disease. How these factors (and perhaps others?) were used to determine the risk level is not explained.

3. *For Berg, Dunbar-Jacob & Sereika's study*

Measure: MDI Chronolog

Type of Reliability or Validity	Value	From present sample?
reliability (reported in literature)	r = .95–.98	yes (r = .95)

Measure: Journal of Daily Asthma Concerns

Type of Reliability or Validity	Value	From present sample?
none provided		no

Measure: Spirometrics Peak-Flow Meter

Type of Reliability or Validity	Value	From present sample?
accuracy	reproducible to ±5%	no

Measure: The Self-Efficacy for Asthma Management Scale

Type of Reliability or Validity	Value	From present sample?
test-retest reliability	.82 at 2 weeks for pilot group .82 at 6 weeks for control group	yes
Cronbach's alpha	ranged from .90 to .82	yes

Measure: The Asthma Self-Management Assessment Tool

Type of Reliability or Validity	Value	From present sample?
test-retest reliability	.42	yes
Cronbach's alpha	.76–.78	yes

For Lewis & colleagues' study

Measure: SvO_2

Type of Reliability or Validity	Value	From present sample?
correlation between *in vivo* and *in vitro* samples	range .89 to .97	no
Cronbach's alpha	can be used for 102 hours with less than a 1% drift for every 24-hour period	no

For Bruce & Grove's study

Measure: Total Serum Cholesterol

Type of Reliability or Validity	Value	From present sample?
Values met the referenced criteria of plus or minus 3% of the true value set by the National Cholesterol Education Program (NCEP)		yes

Measure: LDL

Type of Reliability or Validity	Value	From present sample?
Values met the referenced criteria of plus or minus 3% of the true value set by the National Cholesterol Education Program (NCEP)		yes

Measure: HDL

Type of Reliability or Validity	Value	From present sample?
Values met the referenced criteria of plus or minus 3% of the true value set by the National Cholesterol Education Program (NCEP)		yes

Measure: HDL

Type of Reliability or Validity	Value	From present sample?
No information provided other than the statement that the classification was based on NCEP guidelines. The fact that the guidelines come from the National Heart, Lung, and Blood Institute of NIH provides some degree of content validity.		

4. a. The authors provide no description of the data collection process other than that included in the description of the design and the sample description section.
    b. After informed consent was obtained and randomization status decided, the patient was left undisturbed for 5 minutes lying supine with the head of the bed elevated 20° to 40°. Baseline SvO_2 was recorded at 1-minute intervals during this 5-minute period. The patient was then turned to the left or right lateral position. A single data collector turned the patient and placed two folded standard pillows, one pillow behind the patient's back and one between the patient's knees. For patients in the delayed-backrub group, SvO_2 was again recorded at 1-minute intervals for 5 minutes after the change in body position. The patient was then given a 1-minute backrub. . . Patients assigned to the immediate-backrub group were turned, and the backrub. . . was given immediately. After the backrub, SvO_2 was measured at 1-minute intervals for 5 minutes. There was then a 5-minute period during which 1-minute measurements were made while the patient remained in the lateral position" (p. 135).
    c. The serum lipid values and individual risk factor information were obtained through retrospective medical record review. The greatest threat to the validity of the measures would have been random errors in recording the data from the patient record to a data collection form and then into the computer.
5. a. MDI Chronolog: excellent direct measure of compliance with prescribed use of inhaler.
       Journal of Daily Asthma Concerns: Only measure used from this Diary was the subject report of use of inhaler. This study and previous studies have demonstrated the unreliability of subject report of use.
       Spirometrics peak-flow meter: based on previous literature, this measurement method appears valid and reliable.
       The Self-Efficacy for Asthma Management Scale: reliability for this scale is adequate. There is no information on validity on which to make a judgment.
       The Asthma Self-Management Assessment Tool: Reliability of the instrument is adequate. There is no information on validity on which to make a judgment.
    b. SvO_2 measured using the Explorer continuous venous oximeter is a reliable and valid measurement method.
    c. The measures of lipid levels have acceptable reliability and validity. Although the measure of cardiovascular risk is based on well-accepted guidelines (providing evidence of validity), their application in this study is not sufficiently described to judge reliability. Interrater reliability is not addressed. The authors are not clear about the nonlipid risk factors used in the categorization and the extent to which these are consistent with those recommended by NCEP.

CHAPTER 10
UNDERSTANDING STATISTICS IN RESEARCH

RELEVANT TERMS

Check the glossary in the back of your text for definitions.

KEY TERMS

1. a. Every piece of datum is cross-checked with the original datum for accuracy.
   b. All identified errors are corrected.
   c. Missing points are identified.
   d. Missing data are entered into the data file.
2. You could have listed any three of the following:
   a. Estimates of central tendency are calculated for variables relevant to describing the sample.
   b. Estimates of dispersion are calculated for variables relevant to describing the sample.
   c. Data are examined on each variable using measures of central tendency and dispersion to determine variation in the data and to identify outliers.
   d. Relationships among variables relevant to the sample are examined.
   e. Differences between groups are examined to demonstrate equivalence of study groups.

MAKING CONNECTIONS

Matching Definitions

1. i
2. h
3. f
4. c
5. d
6. e
7. a
8. b
9. g

Categories Categories to Statements

1. b
2. c
3. a
4. d
5. d
6. b
7. d

Significant Differences

Partial-Bed-Test Group Distribution

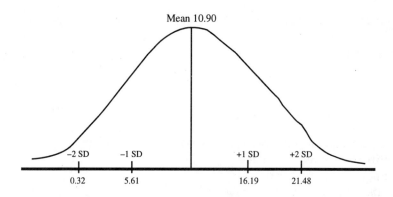

Complete-Bed-Rest Group Distribution

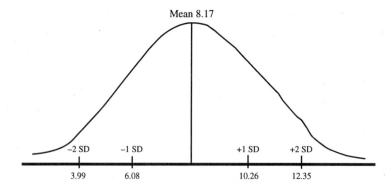

Significance of Results

1. a
2. b
3. a
4. b

PUZZLES

Word Scramble

To be useful, the evidence from data analysis must be carefully examined, organized, and given meaning.

Secret Message

Researchers can never prove things.

Crossword Puzzle

```
[1]S  T  A  T  I  S [2]T  I  C                          [3]E
      T                          [4]M                       X
[5]D  E  C  I  S  I  O  N  T  H  E  O [6]R  Y        O  D     P
   I                          S        E        D        L
[7]I [8]S  I  G [9]N  I  F  I [10]C  A  N  T [11]P  O  W  E  R  [13]P  A
[12]O  M  I  T        O        H        R              N
   P [14]R  E  G  R  E  S  S  I  O  N        E     [15]A  N  O  V  A
   L  I        M              S              S
   I  B        A        [16]D  E  P  E  N  D  E  N  T
[17]C  A  U  S  A  L     C              N           H
   A  T        U  [18]M  E  A  N        T           O
[19]T  A  I  L     U              R  [20]V  A  R  I  A  N  C  E
   I  O     [21]R  A  N  G  E        T
   O  N        V     [22]O  U  T  L  I  E  R  S
   N  [23]M  E  D  I  A  N              V
[24]R  E  S  U  L  T        [25]I  N  F  E  R  E  N  C  E
```

EXERCISES IN CRITIQUE

1.

Variable	Level of Measurement
total serum cholesterol	interval or higher
LDL	interval or higher
HDL	interval or higher
risk level	ordinal—treated as nominal

2. a. t-test
    b. McNemar Test for Significance of Changes
3. a. Before participation in the C.A.R.E. program group
    b. After participation in the C.A.R.E. program group
4. These two groups are dependent The researchers were studying the same subject before and after participation.
5. Given that the level of measurement is interval level or higher, and there are two dependent groups (referred to as paired or matched in the figure), the paired (or dependent) t-test is the appropriate statistical test. No other possible statistical tests are identified by this decision tree. The researchers conducted a separate t-test for each variable. Thus, three t-tests were performed. Use of multiple t-tests causes an escalation of the level of significance, increasing the risk of a Type I error. Using analysis of variance, in which all three variables could be included in one analysis, followed by post hoc tests to identify the significance of specific variables, might have been a better choice.
6. The variable excluded from the analysis was risk level.
7. Risk level was excluded from the analysis because it is an ordinal level measure and is not an appropriate variable for analysis using a t-test.
8. Mean total cholesterol was reduced by 33.82 mg.dl ($t(194) = -16.76$, $p = 0.00$). The results were significant and predicted.
    The mean LDL level was reduced by 28.97 mg/dl ($t(194) = -15.22$, $p = 0.00$). The results were significant and predicted.
    The mean HDL level was increased by 2.75 mg/dl ($t(194) = 3.27$, $p = 0.001$). The results were significant and predicted.
9. a. Before participation in C.A.R.E. group
    b. After participation in C.A.R.E. group
10. According to the decision tree, the recommended analysis for ordinal data is Kruskal-Wallis One-Way Analysis of Variance for Gain Scores. However, the authors treated the risk data as nominal and used the McNemar Test for Significance of Changes. This is a non-parametric analysis that is not described in your textbook. You may find information about it on page 473 of Burns and Grove (1997). The McNemar test uses the chi square symbol (χ^2) as the statistic for the analysis. As a consequence, in a quick examination of the results, it is easy to mistakenly assume that chi square analysis was used.
11. The value obtained from the McNemar test was $\chi^2 > 98.285$, $p = 0.00$. These results are significant and predicted.
12. correlation
13. a. Relationship between cardiovascular risk and total cholesterol level ($r = .67$, $p = .000$; 44% variance explained). This means there is a strong and significant correlation between cardiovascular risk and total cholesterol level. The 44% variance explained is obtained by squaring the r value (r^2) and indicates that 44% of the variation in values of cardiovascular risk and total cholesterol level can be explained by this relationship. However, in considering the meaning of this result, keep in mind that total cholesterol level was used in developing the cardiovascular risk categories. Because of this, the strength of the relationship is overestimated. If one were to remove the effect of total

cholesterol level on classifying cardiovascular risk, the amount of relationship between the two variables would be less.

b. Relationship between cardiovascular risk and LDL cholesterol level (r = .80, p = 0.000; 64% variance explained). This means there is a strong and significant correlation between cardiovascular risk and LDL cholesterol. As in the first relationship discussed, caution is warranted in interpreting this result since LDL cholesterol was used in developing the cardiovascular risk categories and the relationship is probably overestimated.

c. Relationship between cardiovascular risk and HDL cholesterol level (r = −.12; 1.5% of the variance explained). The result is not significant and is unexpected. The authors report that several other studies have found a significant relationship between these two variables. Because HDL was used to develop the risk categories, one would expect to find some degree of relationship between the two variables.

14. a. A significant 13% decrease in the mean total serum cholesterol level occurred after participation in the C.A.R.E. program.

b. A significant 17% reduction in mean LDL levels occurred after participation in the C.A.R.E. program.

c. Mean HDL cholesterol levels significantly increased 5.8% after participation in the C.A.R.E. program.

d. Risk levels were significantly reduced after participation in the C.A.R.E. program. The authors recommend caution in interpreting the results of this analysis. The measurement of risk level in the pretest group was based on the serum lipid profile and the presence of nonlipid risk factors known to affect cardiovascular risk (*e.g.,* exercise, smoking, hypertension, body weight). The measurement of risk level in the posttest group was based only on the serum lipid profile. Other risk factors were not reassessed after participation in the C.A.R.E. program.

The findings stated by the authors are appropriate in relation to the results. Because a comparative descriptive design was used, it is not possible to state that the C.A.R.E. program caused the results. A quasi-experimental design with a comparison or control group would be needed to make that claim. Without a control group, the inference that the program caused the results is unwarranted because there is insufficient evidence that the changes would not have occurred if the program had not been provided.

15. The t-test was appropriate given the level of measurement of the variables. The selection of another analysis strategy such as ANOVA might have reduced the risk of a Type I error from escalation of the level of significance due to the use of repeated t-tests. The use of the McNemar test was acceptable given the level of measurement. Difficulties in interpreting results were due to problems related to the design and measurement, not to the statistical procedures used.

16. "The findings may demonstrate an association between the C.A.R.E. program and the improvements in serum lipid values for the sample."

17. The authors are careful to qualify their conclusion by indicating that the findings may demonstrate an association. This statement is warranted by the data.

18. a. "The results do support the use of educational programs in addition to risk factor assessment in reducing cardiac risk levels."

   b. "Education can be effective in improving lipid profiles and potentially decrease the incidence of CAD (coronary artery disease)."
   c. "Decreasing risk for CAD and the associated loss of productivity, disability, and death could enhance quality of life."
19. The authors walk a narrow line in discussing the implications of their findings while avoiding the assertion that the educational program *caused* the changes they found. The important implication is that there is sufficient evidence that the educational program was effective in reducing risk to warrant quasi-experimental studies to test the cause-effect relationship.
20. This study demonstrates that nurse-managed health education programs such as the C.A.R.E. program can have dramatic impact on people's health and can potentially improve quality of life for high-risk populations.
21. a. educational programs in general
    b. nurse-managed health education programs
22. a. quasi-experimental studies
    b. longitudinal studies
    c. studies using different populations such as minorities, children, and the elderly
    d. cost-benefit analyses

CHAPTER 11
INTRODUCTION TO QUALITATIVE RESEARCH

RELEVANT TERMS
Check the glossary in the back of your text for definitions.

MAKING CONNECTIONS

1.	b	6.	b
2.	a	7.	a
3.	b	8.	b
4.	b	9.	a
5.	a	10.	a

KEY IDEAS

1. Three characteristics of rigor in qualitative research
   a. openness
   b. scrupulous adherence to a philosophical perspective
   c. thoroughness in collecting data
   d. consideration of all the data in the subjective theory development phase
2. You could have listed any three of the following:
   a. The researcher influences the individuals being studied and, in turn, is influenced by them.
   b. The mere presence of the researcher may alter behavior in the setting.
   c. The researcher's personality is a key factor in conducting the study.
   d. The researcher needs to become closely involved in the subject's experience in order to interpret it.
   e. It is necessary for the researcher to be open to the perceptions of the participants, rather than to attach his or her own meaning to the experience.
   f. Individuals being studied often participate in determining research questions, guiding data collection, and interpreting results.
3. You could have listed any four of the following:
   a. coding—developing categories
   b. reflective remarks
   c. marginal remarks
   d. memoing
   e. developing propositions
4. You could have listed any three of the following:
   a. counting
   b. noting patterns, themes
   c. seeing plausibility
   d. clustering
   e. making metaphors
   f. splitting variables
   g. subsuming particulars into the general
   h. factoring
   i. noting relations between variables
   j. finding intervening variables
   k. building a logical chain of evidence
   l. making conceptual/theoretical coherence
5. a. description
   b. analysis
   c. interpretation

Matching qualitative method with characteristics

1. c	6. d
2. b	7. c
3. a	8. b
4. c	9. d
5. a	10. a

CHAPTER 12
CRITIQUING NURSING STUDIES

RELEVANT TERMS

1. i	6. b
2. c	7. e
3. a	8. h
4. j	9. f
5. g	10. d

KEY IDEAS

1. strengths, weaknesses, meaning, and significance
2. You might include any three of the following:
    a. What are the major strengths of the study?
    b. What are the major weaknesses of the study?
    c. Are the findings from the study an accurate reflection of reality?
    d. What is the significance of the findings for nursing?
    e. Are the findings consistent with those for previous studies?
3. You might critique research to share the findings with another health care professional. You might read and critique studies to solve a problem in practice or to summarize research in a topic area for use in practice. You might critique a proposed study to determine if it is ethical to conduct in your clinical agency.
4. a. comprehension
    b. comparison
    c. analysis
    d. evaluation

5. a. descriptive vividness
    b. methodological congruence
    c. analytical preciseness
    d. theoretical connectedness
    e. heuristic relevance

EXERCISES IN CRITIQUE

Conduct the critiques of the studies included in Appendix B of this study guide. Review the answers for the critique exercises for Chapters 3 through 10 to assist you in these critiques. Also ask your instructor to clarify any questions that you might have.

———————————•••••———————————

CHAPTER 13
USING RESEARCH IN NURSING PRACTICE

RELEVANT TERMS

1. e	5. c
2. g	6. h
3. f	7. d
4. a	8. b

KEY IDEAS

1. Research utilization promotes desired outcomes for patients, nurses, and health care agencies. Some of these positive outcomes are identified below.
    a. improve patients' outcomes, such as decrease signs and symptoms of illness, increase function, decrease recovery time, decrease length of hospitalization, increase return-to-work rate, increase satisfaction with care, increase health promotion and illness prevention behaviors.
    b. improve the quality of care
    c. decrease the cost of care
    d. improve the work environment for nurses and promote nurses' productivity.
    e. provide increased access to care by providing different types of health care agencies and services by a variety of health care providers.
2. Obtain the answers to these questions by gathering information in the agencies where you have clinical this semester.

3. You might identify any of the following:
   a. research journals
   b. clinical journals with a major focus on publishing research articles
   c. nursing research conferences
   d. professional nursing meetings and conferences
   e. some collaborative groups of nurses and other health professionals that share research findings
   f. television news reports
   g. newspapers
   h. some popular magazines
   i. agency research newsletters
4. You might identify any of the following:
   a. Axford and Cutchen (1977) developed a preoperative teaching program.
   b. Dracup and Breu (1978) devised a care plan for grieving spouses.
   c. Wichita (1977) developed a program to treat and prevent constipation in nursing home residents.
5. a. identification and synthesis of multiple studies on a selected topic
   b. organization of research knowledge into a solution or clinical protocol for practice
   c. transformation of the clinical protocol into specific nursing actions that are administered to patients
   d. clinical evaluation of the new practice to determine whether it produced the desired outcome
6. You might identify any of the following.
   a. structured preoperative teaching
   b. reducing diarrhea in tube-fed patients
   c. preoperative sensory preparation to promote recovery
   d. preventing decubitus ulcers
   e. intravenous cannula change
   f. closed urinary drainage systems
   g. distress reduction through sensory preparation
   h. mutual goal setting in patient care
   i. clean intermittent catheterization
   j. pain: deliberative nursing interventions
7. a. barriers related to research findings; examples: limited research conducted for certain clinical problems, studies conducted lack replication, limited communication of research findings, and research reports that are complex and difficult to read
   b. barriers created by practicing nurses; examples: practicing nurses do not value research, they are unwilling to read research reports, and they lack the skills to read research reports
   c. barriers created by organizations; examples: some organizations have traditional leadership that is reluctant to change and some organizations neither value research nor provide support for making changes based on research

8. You might include any of the following:
   a. previous practice
   b. felt needs/problems
   c. innovativeness
   d. norms of the social system
9. a. relative advantage
   b. compatibility
   c. complexity
   d. trialability
   e. observability
10. examining the innovation or change for practice and then deciding not to adopt it
11. that the innovation was never seriously considered for use in practice
12. a. Direct application. Description: occurs when an innovation is used exactly as it was developed.
    b. Reinvention. Description: occurs when adopters modify the innovation to meet their own needs.
    c. Indirect effects. Description: occur when nurses incorporate research findings into their knowledge base and use this information to defend a point or to write agency protocols or policies or a clinical paper.
13. a. replacement discontinuance
    b. disenchantment discontinuance
14. a. published integrative reviews of research
    b. published meta-analysis

MAKING CONNECTIONS

1. e
2. c
3. a
4. d
5. b

APPENDIX B

PUBLISHED STUDIES

AN EVALUATION OF A SELF-MANAGEMENT PROGRAM FOR ADULTS WITH ASTHMA

JILL BERG, JACQUELINE DUNBAR-JACOB,
AND SUSAN M. SEREIKA

Approximately 12 million Americans have asthma (National Center for Health Statistics, 1993). Asthma contributes substantially to morbidity and mortality. Indeed, according to National Health Statistics, the death rate attributable to asthma nearly doubled between 1979 and 1987 (National Center for Health Statistics, 1993). Strunk (1989) and other asthma specialists suggest that many of these deaths can be prevented by focusing on the behavioral factors which influence the self-management of asthma.

One component of self-management is compliance with the medical regimen. Noncompliance has been shown to increase mortality and morbidity (Spector et al., 1986). The problem of managing compliance is complicated by the finding that patients overestimate their own compliance with the recommended regimen. Several studies have compared self-report with more direct indicators of medication compliance (Glanz, Stanley, Swartz, & Francis, 1984; Spector et al., 1986). Although patients report approximately 90% compliance, direct measures such as urine testing, electronic monitoring, and pill counts show a 50% to 60% compliance rate (Dunbar, 1980). Thus, interventions aimed at improving compliance need to address the issue of patient's recognition and/or reporting of their regimen behaviors.

Self-management programs encourage the participation of the patient in the daily management of a chronic illness and are based on behavioral and social learning theory (Holroyd & Creer, 1986). Programs which implement self-management strategies have led to less pain in arthritics (Lorig & Holman, 1989), fewer asthma attacks in asthmatics (Creer, 1991), and weight loss in Type II diabetics (Wing, Epstein, Nowalk, & Lamparski, 1986). The addition of a self-efficacy enhancing component to these programs has shown benefit (Lorig & Holman, 1989). Self-efficacy has been shown to be a significant factor for many health care behaviors and is linked to general health functioning (O'Leary, 1985; O'Leary, Shoor, Lorig, & Holman, 1988). It may be postulated that perceived self-efficacy expectancies have a strong influence on chronically ill patients' ability to manage their own care.

The purpose of this study was to evaluate the impact of a nurse-administered asthma self-management program on patient compliance, asthma symptoms, and airway obstruction among patients treated in a rural setting. The majority of studies conducted have targeted urban minority

Author's Note: This study was supported by NINR grant #5-F31NR06787-02 and Glaxo Pharmaceutical grant #NUR005.

populations that are considered more at risk for asthma complications. Few if any studies have considered the rural patient who has a longer distance to travel for care and is dependent for a longer period upon his/her own skills or those of family members during an acute attack. More studies are needed to assess the impact of rural dwelling on those with asthma.

The major hypotheses addressed in this study were that subjects receiving a self-management program would: increase compliance with inhaled medications, decrease the frequency of asthma symptoms, increase the percentage of symptom-free days, and decrease airway obstruction. Secondary hypotheses were that subjects receiving the program would have increased self-efficacy and increased self-management behaviors.

METHOD

Design

This study used a two-group randomized, controlled experimental design. Subjects were randomly assigned to one of two groups: usual care or self-management intervention. Both groups received usual and routine care offered by their physicians. In addition, the experimental group received a 6-week asthma self-management program. Subjects in both groups used the Metered Dose Inhaler (MDI) Chronolog (an electronic measure of inhaler use) daily for 1 week before initiation of the program. Baseline measures were assessed daily for 1 week and included daily peak-flow determinations (using the peak-flow meter and recorded in an asthma diary), compliance with inhaler use (using both the MDI Chronolog and self-report with the diary), asthma symptoms (as self-reported in the diary), and questionnaires to assess asthma self-management and self-efficacy. Treatment consisted of 6 weekly education sessions and self-monitoring throughout the 6-week program. Post-treatment assessments were also made daily for 1 week and were identical to baseline measures.

Sample

The population included rural dwelling adults age 18 years and older with a medical diagnosis of asthma who were being treated with prescribed, regularly administered, inhaled medications other than as-needed bronchodilators. Those who had other respiratory disorders or were current smokers were excluded. After an initial screening for eligibility, subjects were classified according to asthma severity using a three-level severity rating scale—mild, moderate, or severe—based on the American Thoracic Criteria guidelines (National Asthma Education Program Expert Panel Report, 1991). Specific criteria to classify asthma severity included frequency of physical symptoms, work attendance, use of medications, ability to carry out exercise, and peak flow readings. Subjects were stratified on asthma severity due to the possible influence of severity on compliance behavior. A stratified random permuted block scheme was employed for generation of treatment assignments for subjects with moderate and severe asthma (Pocock, 1983; Rudy, Vaska, Daly, Happ, & Shiao, 1993).

Brochures were placed in physician offices and pharmacies, and information about the study was announced on the radio and in newspapers. Potential subjects were called after they indicated an interest in participation. Of 136 adults screened, 87 (64%) were eligible for inclusion. Sixty-eight (78%) signed consent forms were returned. Before the initiation of the program, 13 (19%) withdrew from the study due to weather problems and illness. Therefore, 55 subjects participated in the program with 24 in the control group and 31 subjects in the treatment group. Fifty-four subjects completed the program and 1 subject withdrew but was included in the analysis. No previous intervention studies using similar compliance outcome measures reported the appropriate summary statistics of their data to estimate sample size. In light of this, approximations were made according to recommendations using Cohen (1988). The significance level was set at .05 and the power level was set at .80. A moderate effect size of .5 was chosen, given the nature of the data and lack of pilot data.

The subjects were predominantly female, Caucasian, and married. Subject characteristics are presented in Table 1. The subjects in the sample were relatively well educated. There were no significant differences found between groups on these characteristics.

Procedure

Self-management intervention. The self-management program was adapted from a program designed by Creer, Reynolds, and Kotses (1992) and consisted of 6 sessions, which included information about self-management behaviors and skills, asthma medications, asthma triggers, prevention of asthma attacks, relaxation techniques, psychological responses to asthma, and problem-solving skills. The sessions, which were held in the community, lasted approximately 2 hours and were led by registered nurses who were knowledgeable about asthma. All information that was given to subjects was scripted in a 204-page handbook for group leaders. There were five groups, running from January to May, with approximately 10 subjects in each group. New groups started at 2-week intervals.

Usual care. Subjects randomized to this condition recorded information daily for 1 week following randomization and again at follow-up for treated subjects. No other intervention was given to this group aside from usual care with physician.

Instruments

The instruments used in this study were administered at Week 1 and at Week 7 of each protocol. In order to assure that treatment differences were not due to inability to use the MDI correctly, skills with inhaler use were assessed and reinforced at baseline.

MDI Chronolog. The MDI Chronolog (Forefront Engineering Corporation, Denver, CO) is a monitoring device which is designed to house an MDI and was used to assess compliance. Each time a subject uses the inhaler, a microswitch is activated and the Chronolog records the date and time. Summary output data show the date and time of each subject activation for the period monitored. In this study, this was compared with the self-reported medication prescription.

Table 1. Descriptive Statistics for Treatment and Control Subjects.

CHARACTERISTIC	OVERALL n (%)	TREATMENT n (%)	CONTROL n (%)	χ²(df)*
Gender				
Male	19 (35)	10 (32)	9 (38)	.164(1)
Female	36 (66)	21 (68)	15 (62)	
Ethnicity				
Caucasian	52 (95)	29 (93)	23 (96)	.137(1)
Non-Caucasian	3 (5)	2 (7)	1 (4)	
Marital Status				
Single	19 (35)	11 (35)	8 (33)	.027(1)
Married	36 (65)	20 (65)	16 (67)	
Insurance				
Insured	51 (91)	29 (93)	21 (87)	.599(1)
Not insured	15 (11)	2 (7)	3 (13)	
Education				
Grade school	1 (2)	1 (3)	0 (0)	5.745(3)
High school/some college	35 (64)	23 (74)	12 (50)	
Bachelor's degree	5 (9)	1 (3)	4 (17)	
Graduate school	14 (26)	6 (19)	8 (33)	
Employment				
Full-time/part-time	34 (62)	18 (58)	16 (67)	.424(1)
Unemployed	21 (38)	13 (42)	8 (33)	
Occupation				
Professional	24 (44)	12 (39)	12 (50)	.701(1)
Nonprofessional	31 (56)	19 (61)	12 (50)	
Income (in dollars per year)				
<10,000	9 (17)	6 (20)	3 (12)	2.541(4)
10,001–30,000	20 (37)	13 (43)	7 (29)	
30,001–50,000	11 (20)	5 (17)	6 (25)	
50,001–70,000	7 (13)	3 (10)	4 (17)	
>70,000	7 (13)	3 (10)	4 (17)	
Smoking				
Past	27 (49)	15 (48)	12 (50)	.014(1)
Never	28 (51)	16 (52)	12 (50)	

(continued)

Table 1 (continued). Descriptive Statistics for Treatment and Control Subjects.

CHARACTERISTIC	OVERALL n (%)	TREATMENT n (%)	CONTROL n (%)	$\chi^2(df)*$
Health problems				
Yes	28 (51)	15 (48)	13 (54)	.180(1)
No	27 (49)	16 (52)	11 (46)	
Asthma severity				
Moderate	41 (74)	22 (71)	19 (79)	.479(1)
Severe	14 (26)	9 (29)	5 (21)	
Age				
Mean	50	47	52	
Standard deviation	16	15	15	
t-test				$t = -1.35$
Years with asthma				
Mean	20	17	23	
Standard deviation	17	18	17	
t-test				$t = -1.13$

NOTE: Percentages presented are column percentages.
*$p < .05$.

Compliance scores were calculated for each day and ranged from 0 to 100%. The memory unit of the MDI Chronolog stores the date and time of each triggered activation within approximately 4 seconds. A total of 4,000 events can be stored. Data obtained from the chronolog were downloaded into a computer for storage and analysis. Reliability for the chronolog has been reported in the literature ($r = .95 - .98$) (Rand et al., 1992; Spector et al., 1986) and was tested before initiation of this study ($r = .95$).

Journal of daily asthma concerns. A journal of daily asthma concerns was completed by each subject as part of the self-management program and was also used as an additional measure of compliance for all subjects. This type of diary has been used in self-management programs and other traditional asthma protocols (Creer et al., 1992). Subjects were asked to complete information about medication-taking behavior on a daily basis. For the assessment of asthma symptoms, subjects were required to record information about the presence or absence of four different symptoms: wheeze, cough, shortness of breath, and chest tightness. Subjects also recorded information about the frequency of asthma attacks during daytime and nighttime, and peak-flow readings. Information obtained from the diary on attack frequency was part of a secondary analysis and was not the aim of this study.

Spirometrics peak-flow meter. Subjects were given a peak-flow meter (Spirometric, Inc., Auburn, ME), taught to use it, and asked to record peak-flow measurements twice a day. The peak-flow device is able to measure peak-flow readings of 90–700 lpm for adults. Subjects were instructed to perform three peak-flow measures both in the morning and in the evening and document the highest readings in the asthma diary. Reliability and validity of this tool have been reported (Burns, 1979; Wright & McKerrow, 1959). According to the manufacturer's brochure, the peak-flow meter is accurate and reproducible to ±5%. The peak-flow meters that were used in the study were sent from the factory after manufacture and calibration. A random sample of Spirometric peak-flow meters ($n = 5$) were evaluated for reliability in the respiratory therapy department at the local hospital ($r = .98$).

The Self-Efficacy for Asthma Management Scale. Asthma self-efficacy with inhaled medications was measured by a 14-item Self-Efficacy for Asthma Management Scale (SEAMS), which was developed for this study. The range of possible scores was 0 to 100 with high scores suggesting high self-efficacy. Test-retest reliability was .82 at 2 weeks ($n = 30$) for pilot subjects and .82 at 6 weeks ($n = 24$) for subjects in the control group. Internal consistency ranged from $\alpha = .90$ to $\alpha = .82$.

The Asthma Self-Management Assessment Tool. Asthma self-management was measured by the self-administered Asthma Self-Management Assessment Tool (ASMAT), an adaptation of the Asthma Self-Management Competency Tool developed in 1991 by Taylor et al. The tool contained scenarios for exercise-induced asthma, respiratory tract infections, and a severe asthma attack. Subjects identified their management strategies for each of three types of asthma episodes and were awarded points on the basis of critical incidents and levels of self-management. The self-administered ASMAT had a 6-week test-retest reliability of .42 for control subjects ($n = 24$) with $\alpha = .78$ at Time 1 and $\alpha = .76$ at Time 2. The scores on the ASMAT ranged from 4 to 29. The range of possible scores was 0 to 33 with high scores signifying that subjects indicated that they had the ability to self-manage their asthma during different difficult situations.

Data Analysis

Analysis of covariance with asthma severity as a covariate was the primary statistical procedure used for the analyses of the data. Given the nonnormal distribution of all the compliance data (a J-shaped distribution), the Mann-Whitney U Test was used to test for posttreatment differences in medication compliance between experimental and control groups.

RESULTS

Table 2 presents the baseline and posttreatment measures of central tendency and dispersion for all outcomes. No significant difference between the two groups was observed for compliance at baseline. An examination of posttreatment chronolog compliance revealed a significant difference between the two groups—with the experimental group showing a greater increase

Table 2. Descriptive and Test Statistics for Outcome Variables

OUTCOME	TREATMENT $n = 31$		CONTROL $n = 24$		STAT.* (df)
	PRE	POST	PRE	POST	
Chronolog compliance					
Mean	43	49	40	32	
Standard deviation	29	31	26	28	
Median	40	46	34	23	$U = 271$*
Range	0–100	0–100	0–83	0–88	
Average symptoms per day					
Mean	1.9	1.1	1.2	.85	$F = .284(1)$
Standard deviation	.95	.91	.98	.93	
Median	2.0	1.0	1.1	.57	
Range	0–3.6	0–3.1	0–3.4	0–3.0	
Percentage symptom-free days					
Mean	22	44	43	60	
Standard deviation	30	38	37	37	
Median	13	38	33	64	$U = 282$***
Range	0–100	0–100	0–100	0–100	
Average peak-flow in morning					
Mean	360	359	365	364	$F = .084 (1)$
Standard deviation	105	108	137	142	
Median	351	348	351	342	
Range	150–612	188–700	140–650	250–700	
Average peak-flow in evening					
Mean	347	366	371	381	$F = .000 (1)$
Standard deviation	107	118	140	150	
Median	351	362	340	361	
Range	162–700	207–700	159–669	150–657	

(continued)

Table 2 (continued). Descriptive and Test Statistics for Outcome Variables

OUTCOME	TREATMENT $n = 31$		CONTROL $n = 24$		STAT.* *(df)*
	PRE	POST	PRE	POST	
Asthma self-efficacy					
Mean	58	68	54	64	$F = .104$ (1)
Standard deviation	28	22	21	20	
Median	65	73	51	65	
Range	0–100	0–95	14–100	24–100	
Asthma self-management					
Mean	18	20	18	21	$F = 1.00$ (1)
Standard deviation	6.4	6.2	5.2	5.2	
Median	20	21	19	22	
Range	5–27	4–28	5–26	12–30	

*p < .05.   *** indicates trend p < .1.

in compliance at outcome. However, there was no significant difference for self-reported compliance between the two groups at outcome. As well, no significant difference existed at baseline or posttreatment for the two groups for average total daily symptoms, percentage of symptom-free days, morning or evening peak-flow measurements, self-efficacy, or self-management.

When self-reported compliance and chronolog compliance was examined, median chronolog compliance was 37.5% as compared with a median asthma diary compliance of 93.1%. A modest correlation was documented between the two measures ($r = .44$). Of all subjects, 50% misrepresented their self-reported compliance—which suggests that self-report overestimates compliance with inhaled medications.

DISCUSSION

The findings of this study indicate that subjects who attended the 6-week self-management program increased compliance with inhaled medications compared with subjects receiving usual care. This finding was consistent with other reports of self-management programs in which medication compliance increased after the program (Bailey et al., 1990; Wilson et al., 1993). The use of an electronic monitor made it feasible to evaluate puff spacing. Most manufacturers' package inserts and teaching videos recommend that patients wait at least 1 full minute between puffs. Therefore, the information obtained from this study has important implications for the way in which asthma patients are taught regarding the use of their inhaled medications.

Another relevant finding regarding compliance with inhaled medication concerned the discrepancy between self-report compared with chronolog data. Other studies which examined the use of the chronolog and the asthma diary found that subjects overestimated their compliance behavior compared with the information obtained through the electronic monitor (Coutts, Gibson, & Paton, 1992; Gong, Simmons, Clark, & Tashkin, 1988; Spector et al., 1986; Tashkin et al., 1991). Similarly, in this study, subjects recorded information in their logs that was not corroborated by the chronolog data. Subjects may believe they are complying with inhaler use prescription, which complicates the ability to provide compliance counseling or education in self-management.

The hypothesis that subjects who attended a self-management program would experience a decrease in the frequency of daily asthma symptoms and an increase in the percentage of symptom-free days was not supported by the findings. Several explanations are possible. One is measurement sensitivity: The symptom log may not have had sufficient sensitivity to detect changes in symptom reports. A second explanation may be that the short duration of follow-up was not sufficient to see an effect of alterations in adherence. It may also be that the degree of improvement in adherence was not sufficient to produce a clinical impact. Data do not exist to evaluate the degree of compliance necessary to improve asthma symptoms.

Also, the hypothesis that airway obstruction would decrease with improved compliance was not supported by the findings. Airway obstruction was measured using morning and evening peak-flow readings. It was expected that the increase in compliance with inhaled medications would be accompanied by decreased symptoms and increased peak-flow readings. This finding has been reported elsewhere and there continues to be controversy regarding the sensitivity of peak-flow measurements (Kotses et al., 1991; Wilson et al., 1993).

Neither self-efficacy nor self-management behaviors were modified after the 6-week program. Although each instrument used was stable over time and had good internal consistency, they received limited use. Longitudinal studies that would permit an examination of time to intervention effect would be useful. The self-management programs themselves may need to be revised to target those behaviors that are most problematic for the patient with asthma.

Although the program did not appear to alter self-management behavior as measured by the ASMAT, it had some secondary benefits. Subjects enthusiastic about being included in a study shared many experiences during group meetings concerning the lack of understanding on the part of friends, spouses, and relatives related to the diagnosis of asthma. The ability to problem solve and ventilate feelings of frustration was cited as helpful by study participants. Additionally, subjects had questions about asthma which had not been adequately addressed in busy medical practices in these rural settings. Thus, the supportive problem-solving and educational dimensions were favorably viewed by participants and have implications for clinicians. Education for patients with asthma is necessary but must be targeted to meet specific needs concerning asthma attack prevention and appropriate use of asthma medications. Even after the 6-week program, subjects were confused about which medication to use for an emergency. Nurses can provide asthma patients with information about self-management strategies to ensure appropriate use of medications and decrease morbidity and mortality of these patients.

JILL BERG, Ph.D., R.N., is an associate professor of nursing at California State University, Long Beach. She is currently writing a grant proposal that investigates treatment adherence and self-management issues for adults with asthma.

JACQUELINE DUNBAR-JACOB, Ph.D., R.N., F.A.A.N., is a professor in the Department of Health and Community Systems, School of Nursing and Epidemiology, University of Pittsburgh. She is primarily interested in the field of patient adherence, and is the principal investigator on two grants, one from the Center for Research in Chronic Disorders, NINR, and one on adherence in clinical trials, NHLBI.

SUSAN M. SEREIKA, Ph.D., M.P.H., is an assistant professor and biostatistician in the Department of Health and Community Systems, School of Nursing, and the Departments of Biostatistics and Epidemiology, Graduate School of Public Health, University of Pittsburgh. She is also the director of research support care for the Center for Research in Chronic Disorders. Her research focuses on statistical modeling of longitudinal data.

References

BAILEY, W.C., RICHARDS, J.M., BROOKS, C.M., SOONG, S., WINDSOR, R.A., & MANZELLA, B.A. (1990). A randomized trial to improve self-management practices of adults with asthma. *Archives of Internal Medicine, 150,* 1664–1668.

BURNS, K. (1979). An evaluation of two inexpensive instruments for assessing airway flow. *Annals of Allergy, 43,* 246–249.

COHEN, L. (1988). *Statistical power analysis for the behavioral sciences.* New York: Academic Press.

COUTTS, J.A.P., GIBSON, N.A., & PATON, J.Y. (1992). Measuring compliance with inhaled medication in asthma. *Archives of Diseases of the Child, 67,* 332–333.

CREER, T.L. (1991). The application of behavioral procedures to childhood asthma: Current and future perspectives. *Patient Education and Counseling, 17,* 9–22.

CREER, T.L., REYNOLDS, R.V.C., & KOTSES, H. (1992). *A Handbook for Asthma Self-Management by Adults.* Athens: Ohio University Press.

DUNBAR, J. (1980). Adhering to medical advice: A review. *International Journal of Mental Health, 9,* 70–87.

GLANZ, K., STANLEY, B., SWARTZ, M., & FRANCIS, M. (1984). Compliance with an experimental drug regimen for treatment of asthma: Its magnitude, importance and correlates. *Journal of Chronic Disease, 37,* 815–824.

GONG, H., SIMMONS, M., CLAR, V., & TASHKIN, D. (1988). Metered dose inhaler usage in subjects with asthma: Comparison of Nebulizer Chronolog and daily diary record information. *Journal of Allergy and Clinical Immunology, 82,* 5–10.

HOLROYD, K.A., & CREER, T.L. (1986). *Self-Management of Chronic Disease.* New York: Academic Press.

KOTSES, H., STOUT, C., WIGAL, J.K., CARLSON, B., CREER, T.L., & LEWIS, P. (1991). Individualized asthma self-management: A beginning. *Journal of Asthma, 28*(4), 287–289.

LORIG, K., & HOLMAN, H.R. (1989). Long term outcomes of an arthritis self-management study: Effects of reinforcement efforts. *Social Science Medicine, 29,* 221–224.

NATIONAL CENTER FOR HEALTH STATISTICS (1993). *National Heart, Lung, and Blood Institute Data Fact Sheet* (National Health Interview Survey Publication No. ASI 4476–81.). Washington, DC: U.S. Government Printing Office.

NATIONAL ASTHMA EDUCATION PROGRAM EXPERT PANEL REPORT (1991). *Executive Summary: Guidelines for the diagnosis and management of asthma* (DHHS Publication No. 91–3042A) Bethesda, Maryland: National Institutes of Health.

O'LEARY, A. (1985). Self-efficacy and health behavior. *Respiratory Therapy, 23,* 437–451.

O'LEARY, A., SHOOR, S., LORIG, K., & HOLMAN, H.R. (1988). A cognitive behavioral treatment for rheumatoid arthritis. *Health Psychology, 7,* 527–544.

POCOCK, S.L. (1983). *Clinical Trials: A Practical Approach.* New York: John Wiley.

RAND, C.S., WISE, R.A., NIDES, M., SIMMONS, M.S., BLEECKER, E.R., KUSEK, H.W., LI, V.C., & TASHKIN, D.P. (1992). Metered-dose inhaler adherence in a clinical trial. *American Review of Respiratory and Critical Care Medicine, 146,* 1559–1564.

RUDY, E.B., VASKA, P.L., DALY, B.J., HAPP, M.B., & SHIAO, P. (1993). Permuted block design for randomization in a nursing clinical trial. *Nursing Research, 42,* 287–289.

SPECTOR, S.L. KINSMAN, R., MAWHINNEY, H., SIEGEL, S.C., RACHELEFSKY, G.S., KATZ, R.M., & ROHR, A.H. (1986). Compliance of patients with asthma with an experimental aerosolized medication: Implications for controlled clinical trials. *Journal of Allergy Clinical Immunology, 77,* 65–70.

STRUNK, R.C., (1989). Death caused by asthma: Minimizing the risks. *Journal of Respiratory Diseases, 10*(3), 21–36.

TASHKIN, D.P., RAND, C., NIDES, M., SIMMONS, M., WISE, R., COULSON, A.H., LI, V., & GONG, H. (1991). A nebulizer chronolog to monitor compliance with inhaler use. *American Journal of Medicine, 91*(supp. 4A), 33S–36S.

TAYLOR, G.H., REA, H.H., McNAUGHTON, S., SMITH, L., MULDAR, J., ASHER, M.I., MITCHELL, E.A., SEELVE, E., & STEWART, A.W. (1991). A tool for measuring the asthma self-competency of families. *Journal of Psychosomatic Research, 35,* 483–491.

WILSON, S.R., SCAMAGAS, P., GERMAN, D.F., HUGHES, G.W., LULLA, S., COSS, S., CHARDON, L., THOMAS, R.G., STARR-SCHNEIDKRAUT, N., STANCAVAGE, F.B., & ARSHAM, G.M. (1993). A controlled trial of two forms of self-management education for adults with asthma. *American Journal of Medicine, 94,* 564–576.

WING, R.R., EPSTEIN, L.H., NOWALK, M.P., & LAMPARSKI, D. (1986). Behavioral self-regulation in the treatment of patients with diabetes mellitus. *Psychological Bulletin, 99,* 78–89.

WRIGHT, B.M., & McKERROW, C.B. (1959). Maximum forced expiratory flow rate as a measure of ventilatory capacity. *British Medical Journal, 2,* 1041.

THE EFFECT OF TURNING AND BACKRUB ON MIXED VENOUS OXYGEN SATURATION IN CRITICALLY ILL PATIENTS

Patricia Lewis, Eva Nichols, Gloria Mackey, Anecita Fadol, Lorinda Sloane, Evangelina Villagomez, and Patricia Liehr

• *Objective: To examine the effect of a change in body position (right or left lateral) and timing of backrub (immediate or delayed) on mixed venous oxygen saturation in surgical ICU patients.*

• *Methods: A repeated-measures design was used to study 57 critically ill men. Mixed venous oxygen saturation was recorded at 1-minute intervals for 5 minutes in each of three periods: baseline, after turning, and after backrub. Subjects were randomly assigned to body position and timing of the backrub. Subjects in the immediate-backrub group were turned and given a 1-minute backrub. Mixed venous oxygen saturation was measured at 1-minute intervals for 5 minutes at two points: after the backrub and then with the patient lying on his side. For subjects in the delayed-backrub group, saturation was measured at 1-minute intervals for 5 minutes at two different points: after the subject was turned to his side and after the backrub.*

• *Results: Both position and timing of backrub had significant effects on mixed venous oxygen saturation across conditions over time. Subjects positioned on their left side had a significantly greater decrease in saturation when the backrub was started. At the end of the backrub, saturation was significantly lower in subjects lying on their left side than in subjects lying on their right side. The pattern of change differed according to the timing of the backrub, and return to baseline levels of saturation after intervention differed according to body position.*

• *Conclusions: Two consecutive interventions (change in body position and backrub) cause a greater decrease in mixed venous oxygen saturation than the two interventions separated by a 5-minute equilibrium period. Turning to the left side decreases oxygen saturation more than turning to the right side does. Oxygen saturation returns to clinically acceptable ranges within 5 minutes of an intervention. In patients with stable hemodynamic conditions, the standard practice of turning the patient and immediately giving a backrub is recommended. However, it is prudent to closely monitor individual patterns of mixed venous oxygen saturation, particularly in patients with unstable hemodynamic conditions.*

Backrubs and changes in body position are established interventions for enhancing patients' comfort, mobilizing pulmonary secretions, and improving tissue perfusion through pressure reduction.[1] Understanding the best strategies for combining these interventions may improve patients' outcomes and make the best use of nursing time.

BACKGROUND

Patients are commonly repositioned to the supine, right lateral, and left lateral positions before a backrub. The physiological effect of these interventions is questioned only if untoward changes are noted. Vital signs are routinely used to assess patients' responses to interventions such as changes in position and backrubs. Another useful measurement is mixed venous oxygen saturation (SvO_2), an indicator of oxygen delivery and consumption.

Normally, patients are given a backrub immediately after a change in body position. The consequences of multiple, sequential activities can be hemodynamic compromise. We were interested in comparing the effects on SvO_2 of turning with an immediate backrub and turning with a delayed backrub. The following research questions were addressed:

1. Does the change in SvO_2 after a 1-minute backrub in critically ill patients given the backrub immediately after turning differ from the change in SvO_2 in patients given the backrub 5 minutes after turning?
2. What is the effect of right and left lateral positions on SvO_2 in critically ill patients?

FRAMEWORK FOR THE STUDY

This study is based on the physiological principles underlying SvO_2. The SvO_2 indirectly reflects the balance between oxygen supply and tissue oxygen demands.[2-4] The normal range of SvO_2 is 60% to 80%. Determinants of SvO_2 are arterial oxygen saturation (SaO_2), hemoglobin levels, cardiac output, and tissue oxygen demands. Therefore, an uncompensated reduction in SaO_2, hemoglobin level, or cardiac output or increases in tissue oxygen consumption will result in a decreased SvO_2.[3]

The SaO_2 influences the SvO_2. Pathological pulmonary conditions that impair oxygen transfer at the alveolar-capillary membrane will result in less oxygen available for transport through the circulation. In addition, a deficit in hemoglobin reduces the oxygen-binding capacity of the blood and affects oxygen supply to the tissues. The cardiac output is the means for transporting oxyhemoglobin through the system. The fourth factor that influences SvO_2 is tissue oxygen demand. Tissue extraction of oxygen is increased in conditions such as fever, seizures, and shivering. Routine nursing care such as turning the patient, suctioning, weighing, bed baths, and backrubs may cause increased oxygen consumption. Rather than indicating a specific clinical event, SvO_2 reflects the balance between oxygen supply and demand. SvO_2 trends must be monitored closely to maximize medical and nursing intervention to optimize oxygenation and prevent an imbalance between oxygen supply and demand.[2-4]

LITERATURE REVIEW

Patients in the critical care environment are subject to conditions that may affect oxygen delivery and increase oxygen demand. Routine nursing interventions thought to be beneficial in preventing untoward outcomes may cause an imbalance between oxygen supply and demand. Investigators have studied the effects of a limited number of nursing activities on SvO_2 values. Body positioning has been the focus of much research[5-8] and has been a variable examined when other interventions such as bathing[9] and backrub[10] have been studied.

Shively[5] examined the effects of changes in body position and frequency of the changes on oxygenation in 30 subjects. Patients were randomly assigned to one of two groups. Patients in one group were turned every hour, whereas those in the other group were turned every 2 hours. All patients were turned in the following sequence: right lateral with the head of the bed elevated 20°, supine with the head of the bed at 45°, left lateral with the head of the bed at 20°, and supine with the head of the bed at 20°. SvO_2 values were recorded immediately after the turn (baseline values) and at 15 minutes, 1 hour, and 2 hours (second group only) after each change in position. The results showed no significant difference in SvO_2 between the two groups for time of turning ($P = .5757$) or for the four variations in body position ($P = .1351$). The difference in mean SvO_2 values measured at baseline and at 15 minutes after the turn was significant ($P = .0001$). There was also a significant difference between baseline values and the values determined 1 hour after changes in position ($P = .0001$). Interaction between position and time of measurement was significant (multivariate test: $F[6,23] = 6.87, P = .0003$; univariate test: $P = .0001$). Mean SvO_2 values were lowest immediately after a turn to the left lateral position.

Tidwell et al.[6] studied the effect of six position changes on 34 patients 4 to 8 hours after coronary artery bypass surgery. The initial change for all subjects was from supine to 30° head-of-bed elevation and back to supine. Thereafter, patients were randomized into two sequences: (1) right lateral, supine, left lateral, and then supine or (2) left lateral, supine, right lateral, and then supine. Subjects maintained each position for 30 minutes. SvO_2, SaO_2, and oxygen consumption were recorded simultaneously immediately before the position change, at each minute after the position change for 5 minutes, and at 15 and 25 minutes. Significant decreases in SvO_2 occurred with all changes from lateral and return to supine: supine to 45° right lateral recumbent ($P = .0$), 45° right lateral recumbent to supine ($P = .0002$), supine to 45° left lateral recumbent ($P = .0$), and 45° left lateral recumbent to supine ($P = .0031$). The greatest difference in mean SvO_2 values occurred in the interval between the time immediately before the change in position and the first minute after the change. Moving from supine to the right lateral recumbent position resulted in a decrease in mean SvO_2 of 6.1% whereas moving from supine to the left lateral recumbent position decreased SvO_2 by 5.6%.

Winslow et al.[7] studied the effect of change in body position in 174 patients as part of a multiinterventional study. All patients had pulmonary artery catheters in place. The subjects rested for 10 minutes and then were placed in the right or left side-lying position with the head of the bed at 20° and a pillow supporting them at a 60° angle from the bed. SvO_2 and heart rate were measured immediately after the turn and then at 1-minute intervals for 4 minutes. The decision to obtain the measurements with the subject in the right or left side-lying position was determined by the location of the tip of the subject's pulmonary artery catheter. Because the catheter tip was located in the right pulmonary artery in 85% of the subjects, only 15% of subjects were turned to the left side-lying position. Mean SvO_2 decreased from 67 ±8% at baseline to 61 ±10% ($P <.0001$) immediately after turning and gradually returned to 66 ±8% ($P <.002$) within 4 minutes. The decrease in SvO_2 immediately after turning was a change of 9% from baseline, which was more marked than the decrease in SvO_2 after other interventions. Analysis showed no significant difference in SvO_2 between subjects turned to the right and subjects turned to the left.

Copel and Stolarik[8] studied the effect of turning on 11 subjects after elective coronary artery bypass surgery. The majority of patients were turned from supine to the right lateral position and stayed in the lateral position for 6 to 16 minutes. SvO_2 decreased a mean of 11% immediately after the change in position. The difference in SvO_2 values obtained before and after turning was significant ($t = 9.87$, $df = 10$, $P <.01$) and persisted for a mean of 7.5 minutes.

Atkins et al.[9] studied the effect on SvO_2 of the timing of a bed bath in 30 subjects less than 24 hours after coronary artery bypass surgery. The study involved two bed baths consisting of a bathing phase and a turning phase early (mean, 3.6 hours) and late (mean, 18.5 hours) in the immediate postoperative period. Mean SvO_2 decreased from baseline values during the early and late bed baths by 1.6% and 1.9%, respectively. The mean SvO_2 during the turning phase decreased 9.2% and 12.1% from baseline, respectively. The return to baseline SvO_2 value after intervention required 3 to 4 minutes.

Tyler et al[10] studied the effect of a 1-minute backrub on SvO_2 and heart rate in 173 critically ill patients as a part of the multiinterventional study[7] previously discussed. The backrub was the third intervention. All patients were placed supine, and baseline SvO_2 and heart rate were measured. The subjects were then turned to a lateral position. As previously described, the direction of the turn was determined by the location of the tip of the pulmonary artery catheter. The side-lying position was maintained for 15 minutes before the 1-minute backrub. Data were collected immediately after the backrub and then at 1-minute intervals for 4 minutes. After the backrub, mean SvO_2 decreased immediately from 67%, the baseline value, to 63% ($P = .0001$). SvO_2 returned to baseline within 4 minutes.

In summary, nursing interventions cause a significant decrease in SvO_2 immediately after the intervention is started. SvO_2 values usually return to baseline within 3 to 9 minutes, depending on the intervention.

METHODS

An experimental, repeated-measures, nested design was used. The study was approved by the institutional review board, and all subjects signed an informed consent document. Subjects were randomly assigned to right or left lateral position and then to an immediate or a delayed backrub. The sealed-envelope technique was used to assign position and then timing of backrub.

Sample and Setting

A convenience sample of 57 critically ill men in a surgical ICU at the Veterans Affairs Medical Center, Houston, Tex, was studied. No women were included in the sample because of the population of the study site. Power analysis[11] for repeated measures indicates that 23 subjects are needed to detect a medium effect at the .05 level of significance with a power of 0.80 and an estimated mean correlation among the repeated measures of 0.50 when only seven repeated measures are collected. This study had two grouping variables: position and immediacy of backrub. A minimum of 23 subjects was recruited into each group. This sample size provided more than adequate power, because 15 repeated measures were recorded for each subject.[11]

Subjects who had a fiber-optic pulmonary artery catheter in place, a baseline SvO_2 of 50% or higher, and an indwelling arterial catheter with normal waveform were eligible for inclusion in the study. Exclusion criteria included age less than 18 years, sepsis, pneumonectomy or lobectomy, mechanical assist devices in place, organ transplantation, and use of neuromuscular blocking agents. No subjects were excluded because of advanced age.

Instrumentation

Patients had fiber-optic thermodilution pulmonary artery catheters (the Explorer continuous venous oximeter, American Edwards Laboratories, Irvine, Calif) in place to measure SvO_2. Researchers have compared SvO_2 values obtained with fiber-optic thermodilution pulmonary artery catheters (in vivo) with values obtained in laboratory analyses (in vitro). For critically ill patients, correlations between in vivo and in vitro samples ranged from .89 to .97.[12-14] In addition to these high correlations, Baele et al.[12] found, in a sample of critically ill adults, that the catheters could be used for 102 hours with less than a 1% drift for every 24-hour period. Calibration of each catheter was completed within 24 hours before data collection.

Procedure

After informed consent was obtained and randomization status decided, the patient was left undisturbed for 5 minutes lying supine with the head of the bed elevated 20° to 40°. Baseline SvO_2 was recorded at 1-minute intervals during this 5-minute period (Figure 1).

The patient was then turned to the left or right lateral position. A single data collector turned the patient and placed two folded standard pillows, one pillow behind the patient's back and one between the patient's knees. For patients in the delayed-backrub group, SvO_2 was again recorded at 1-minute intervals for 5 minutes after the change in body position. The patient was then given a 1-minute backrub. The backrub procedure was as follows:

1. The nurse poured lotion into his or her hands and warmed it by rubbing the hands together.

2. With lotion on both hands and palms flat and side by side, the nurse rubbed the patient's sacrum slowly in a circular motion for three circles.

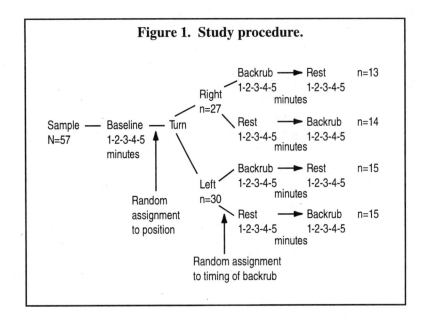

Figure 1. Study procedure.

3. The nurse then moved his or her hands slowly up the medial aspect of the patient's back and stopped at the scapular level.

4. Three circular motions were done in this region.

5. The nurse then moved his or her hands down the lateral aspect of the patient's back to massage the areas of the right and left iliac crests for three circular motions.

At the end of the backrub, one pillow was positioned behind the patient's back and one between the patient's knees, and SvO_2 was recorded from a digital readout at 1-minute intervals for 5 minutes.

Patients assigned to the immediate-backrub group were turned, and the backrub, as just described, was given immediately. After the backrub, SvO_2 was measured at 1-minute intervals for 5 minutes. There was then a 5-minute period during which 1-minute measurements were made while the patient remained in the lateral position.

Subjects

The mean age of the subjects was 60.9 years (standard deviation [SD] = 8.6; range, 40–79 years). Forty-nine subjects had had aortocoronary bypass surgery; 6, resection of an aortic aneurysm; 1, atrial septal repair; and 1, an esophogastrectomy. All subjects were in the surgical ICU at the time of the intervention. Forty-nine subjects were receiving oxygen by either face mask ($n = 22$) or nasal cannula ($n = 27$). Four subjects were receiving mechanical ventilation; 3 of these were receiving 5 cm of positive end-expiratory pressure. The remaining 4 subjects had no supplemental oxygen therapy. Mean SaO$_2$, hemoglobin level, cardiac output, and cardiac index are given in Table 1. Mean baseline heart rate for the sample was 98 beats per minute (SD = 15). There was no significant difference in the factors (SaO$_2$, hemoglobin level, or cardiac output) affecting oxygen supply or heart rate for the position group or the immediacy-of-backrub group. Table 2 lists the distribution of vasoactive therapies for the study subjects. Subjects receiving dopamine or IV nitroglycerin were equally distributed across groups (position or immediacy of backrub) as determined by chi-square analysis ($P > .05$). For all patients receiving dopamine, the dosage of the drug was a renal perfusion dosage and was not being titrated. Twenty-nine subjects were assigned to receive a delayed backrub; 28, an immediate backrub.

Table 1. Means and standard deviations for factors affecting oxygen supply.

FACTOR	MEAN	SD
SaO$_2$ (%)	97.5	2.0
Hemoglobin (g/L)	89	12
Cardiac output (L/min)	6.6	1.2
Cardiac index (L/min per m^2)	3.23	0.58

Table 2. Number of subjects receiving vasoactive therapy.

	No. OF SUBJECTS	
MEDICATION	RECEIVING THERAPY	NOT RECEIVING THERAPY
Dopamine	39	18
Dobutamine	3	54
Norepinephrine	2	55
Epinephrine	1	56
Nitroprusside	1	56
Nitroglycerin	33	24

Data Analysis

Data were analyzed by using a 2 × 2 × 3 × 5 repeated-measures analysis of variance. The first two factors were grouping factors: (1) timing of backrub: immediate or delayed and (2) position: right or left. The second two factors were repeated measures factors: (1) condition: baseline, back-rub, rest, and (2) time: 1 through 5 minutes. SvO$_2$ was the dependent measure. Greenhouse-Geisser adjusted degrees of freedom were used when appropriate. Scheffé tests (P < .05) were used to indicate significant differences between levels of SvO$_2$ at specific times during the protocol.

RESULTS

Both position ($F = 3.78$, $P = .007$) and immediacy of backrub ($F = 8.1$, $P = .000$) had significant effects on SvO$_2$ across conditions over time.

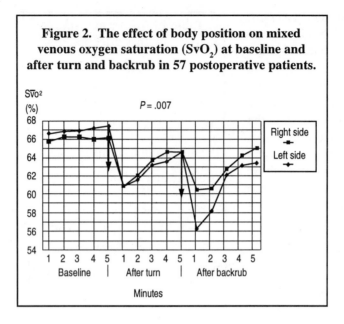

Figure 2. The effect of body position on mixed venous oxygen saturation (SvO$_2$) at baseline and after turn and backrub in 57 postoperative patients.

Except for the subjects who were on their left side for the backrub, when an intervention was introduced, (the turn itself or the beginning of the backrub), SvO$_2$ decreased significantly and then returned to baseline levels within 5 minutes as the condition persisted (Figure 2). Subjects positioned on their left side had a significantly greater (Scheffé tests, $P < .05$) decrease in SvO$_2$ when the backrub was initiated than subjects positioned on their right side (left side: mean = 64.6%, SD 6.7 to mean = 56.3%, SD 7.4; right side: mean 64.6%, SD = 8.9 to mean = 60.5%, SD = 11.2). At the end of the backrub, SvO$_2$ was significantly lower (Scheffé tests, $P < .05$) in subjects on their left side (mean = 63.4%, SD 7.2) than in subjects on their right side (mean = 65.0%, SD = 9.1). Further, for subjects on their left side, the final reading after the backrub was significantly lower than the final baseline value (Scheffé tests, $P < .05$). These lower SvO$_2$ values during the backrub occurred even though subjects lying on their left side had significantly higher (Scheffé tests, $P < .05$) values at baseline than subjects lying on their right side did.

Subjects who had an immediate backrub had a significant decrease in SvO$_2$ (Scheffé tests, $P < .05$ when they were turned and the backrub was started (from mean = 65.9%, SD = 8.0 to mean = 56.7%, SD = 10.9). In this condition, the interventions (turn and backrub) occurred together. Steady increases in SvO$_2$ occurred during the backrub and continued into the control condition (Figure 3), during which the subject remained positioned on his side. In contrast, subjects who had a delayed backrub had significant decreases (Scheffé tests, $P < .05$) in SvO$_2$ both when turned (from mean = 67.7%, SD = 6.8 to mean = 58.8%, SD 7.6) and when the

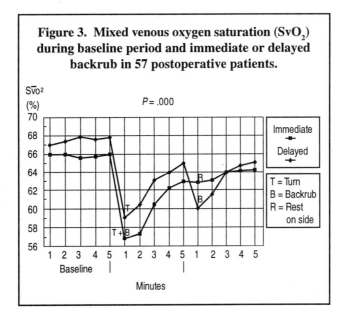

Figure 3. Mixed venous oxygen saturation (SvO$_2$) during baseline period and immediate or delayed backrub in 57 postoperative patients.

backrub was started (from mean 64.9%, SD 7.2 to mean 60.0%, SD = 7.7; Figure 3). SvO$_2$ increased during the 5 minutes after the introduction of each intervention. Therefore, the pattern of SvO$_2$ change was affected by the immediacy of the backrub.

DISCUSSION

Changes in Body Position

Although positioning to the right or left side is implicit in many nursing interventions, few studies have systematically studied the effect on SvO$_2$ of lying on the right or the left side. Shively[5] was the first to investigate this phenomenon. Two years after Shively's report, Tidwell et al.[6] reported another systematic investigation of the effect of positioning on oxygen delivery and utilization.

We systematically examined the effects of positioning on SvO$_2$ as a secondary research question. In the two previous investigations, all subjects were studied in both right and left lateral positions. In our study, subjects were randomly assigned to the right or the left lateral position. By itself, turning onto either side did not result in different SvO$_2$ values for the two groups (Figure 2). However, the combination of a turn to the left side plus a backrub produced the greatest decrease in SvO$_2$. The difference from the baseline SvO$_2$ was significant and persisted 5 minutes after the backrub.

The changes associated with positioning only are most like those reported by Tidwell et al.,[6] who found similar differences in SvO_2 when subjects were turned to the right or left side (6.1% decrease for turn to right and 5.6% decrease for turn to left). In our study, SvO_2 decreased 5.2% for a turn to the right and 6.4% for a turn to the left. Both our findings and those of Tidwell et al. contrast with the results of Shively,[5] who found that the lowest SvO_2 values occurred after a turn to the left side. Shively found a mean decrease of 7.7% (from 68.5% to 60.8%) in SvO_2 when subjects were positioned on their right side and a mean decrease of 11.1% (from 68.5% to 57.4%) when they were positioned on their left side. It is difficult to synthesize these different findings. At best, one can conclude that SvO_2 will decrease when a patient is turned, regardless of the side to which the patient is turned. In our study, 25 (44%) of the 57 subjects had SvO_2 values less than 60% associated with the turn. The lowest SvO_2 value was 47%, decreasing from a baseline of 52%. This subject's SvO_2 returned to 50% within 1 minute and was 52% at the end of the protocol. It is important to continue to assess individual SvO_2 values when patients are turned. The quick rebound of SvO_2 values noted in our study leads to questions about the clinical significance of the decrease in SvO_2 value to less than 60%. Even when mean values decreased into the 50% range, they did not remain that low for more than 3 minutes (Figure 2).

The most significant decreases in SvO_2 associated with turning occurred in subjects turned on their left side and given a backrub. This finding is difficult to explain on the basis of physiological parameters, because a backrub is a passive activity that demands no additional energy. Possibly, the left-sided position was associated with more pain. We did not collect data on the positioning of chest tubes, but evaluation of such data could add valuable information. If most chest tubes were positioned on the left side, the subtle added movements associated with a backrub might have exaggerated discomfort associated with positioning. Because the majority of patients were extubated at the time data were collected, it is expected that painful discomfort would have led to a request to be withdrawn from the study. No subjects asked to be withdrawn.

Although a significant difference persisted between baseline SvO_2 values (mean = 67.4%, SD = 7.4) and values obtained 5 minutes after the backrub (mean 63.4%, SD 7.2), this difference was not clinically important. Once again, although the mean values are within clinically acceptable limits, individual patterns of changes in SvO_2 should be closely assessed.

Immediacy of Backrub

In clinical practice, patients are turned, and backrubs are given. The most likely result of this sequence is that the patient actually gets a backrub. If the nurse leaves the patient and returns later for the backrub, intervening activities decrease the likelihood that a backrub will occur. Therefore, the question of when to give a backrub to facilitate optimal oxygen delivery and consumption and simultaneously conserve nursing time becomes important. In the delayed-backrub group, mean SvO_2 decreased from 64.9% to 60.0%. This change is not considered clinically significant, because the SvO_2 remained within the normal range. This reduction in SvO_2 may have been due to the combination of (1) the removal of the pillows, an intervention that includes a component of turning or repositioning; and (2) stimulation from the backrub. This result is similar to the findings in the study of Tyler et al.,[10] in which SvO_2 decreased significantly with the backrub even after a period of nonintervention. Interestingly, in our study, in 9 of the 25 subjects who had SvO_2 values less than 60% with the change in body position, initiation of the backrub increased the SvO_2 values. Four of the 9 had SvO_2 values greater than 60% with the start of the backrub. Three of these 4 were characterized by the recorder as very drowsy, very relaxed, or showing comfortable "moaning" during the backrub.

Two subjects had SvO_2 values that decreased to 33% with the backrub. Both subjects were in the immediate-backrub group. Their baseline SvO_2 values were 55% and 56%. One was positioned on his left side; the other, on the right side. The recorder stated that one of the patients was very tense (bearing down, grunting, holding breath). Both patients were extubated, alert, and receiving low-dose dopamine and nitroglycerin. The tense subject's SvO_2 returned to 53% in 4 minutes and to 56% after the additional 5 minutes in the side-lying position. The other subject's baseline SvO_2 was 52%. This subject's SvO_2 was 48% at 4 minutes after the turn to his right side and a backrub and 50% after the additional 5 minutes in the side-lying position. Cardiac output, cardiac index, and SaO_2 were within normal range for both subjects. The hemoglobin levels were 8.5 and 7.7 g/dL (85 and 77 g/L).

Six patients had an SvO_2 of 44% to 49% immediately after the backrub. Five of the six were in the immediate-backrub group. In two of the six, SvO_2 values were within normal limits by the end of the protocol. In the other four subjects, the SvO_2 values increased to 52% to 56% by the end of the protocol. The recorder stated that all four patients were tense, moaning, talking, coughing, or not comfortable. These behaviors may have increased oxygen consumption and limited the SvO_2 rebound seen in other subjects.

These examples show that multiple consecutive interventions may result in an even more significant decrease in SvO_2 for particular subjects. Atkins et al.[9] compared SvO_2 in patients having a continuous or an interrupted bed bath and concluded that consecutive interventions may have cumulative effects. For example, bathing the anterior surface of a patient's body is associated with minimal exertion by the patient, whereas turning the patient causes a significant decrease in SvO_2, and coughing, shivering, and agitation with activity such as turning can decrease the SvO_2 even more severely. Critically ill patients often require endotracheal suctioning, a procedure that can cause coughing or agitation. For comfort, patients may be turned to a lateral position after the suctioning and given a backrub. In this real-world example, patients are at risk for deterioration in their condition, especially if their baseline status was unstable. In our study, the mean SvO_2 decreased to 56.7% with the combined activity of a change in body position and a backrub. This decrease was not clinically significant. If the SvO_2 is 50% or less, oxygen delivery is marginal for oxygen demands, a situation that could cause deterioration in the patient's clinical condition, and possibly death.[4] We do not mean that the SvO_2 should be less than 50%; rather, a momentary decrease in SvO_2 will be outweighed by the benefits of the intervention (e.g., suctioning, turning, backrub).

Our results do not support the approach of Tyler et al.[10] of waiting 15 minutes between turning the patient and given the backrub. Rather, we suggest that the standard practice of turning the patient and immediately giving a backrub be retained. The type of activity will determine the effect of multiple consecutive interventions on SvO_2. The less the exertion, the more likely it is that the patient will tolerate combined interventions. SvO_2 returned to baseline within 5 minutes of an intervention in most studies.[5–7,9,10,15] Copel and Stolarik[8] found that it took 7.5 minutes for subjects' SvO_2 to return to baseline values. In our study, SvO_2 immediately started to increase after an intervention but did not consistently return to baseline values within 5 minutes. The slower return occurred when subjects were on their left side. Although SvO_2 did not reach baseline values, mean SvO_2 did return to clinically acceptable levels within 5 minutes.

Generalizability of Findings

Several investigators[7,9,10] have studied factors that influence SvO_2, for example, SaO_2, hemoglobin level, cardiac output, and cardiac index. The reported values, like those of our study, were within normal limits. However, the mean hemoglobin level in subjects in our study was 89 g/L (SD = 12), whereas the mean in previous studies was 110 g/L. Our study was done in a time when blood products were given more judiciously than they had been in earlier times. Generally, the reported values of the factors that influence SvO_2 confirm the hemodynamic stability of the study populations, as do data on baseline SvO_2.

In all studies,[5–10] patients had mean baseline SvO_2 values within normal limits. In our study, the mean baseline SvO_2 was 66.0% to 67.8%. In only 8 (14%) of 57 subjects were baseline SvO_2 values less than 60%. The lowest baseline SvO_2 was 50%. Therefore our findings and those of other studies can be generalized only to a population of postoperative patients with hemodynamically stable conditions. During the past 5 years, SvO_2 monitoring has increasingly been used for patients with unstable hemodynamic conditions. The database that currently guides nursing intervention relative to oxygen delivery and consumption was developed with patients who had a stable hemodynamic status. The database should now be tested in patients with less stable conditions for whom SvO_2 monitoring is the current standard of care. The effects of these interventions most likely would be more dramatic in these compromised patients.

Implications for Practice

We recommend continuing the current practice of turning the patient and administering a backrub immediately in patients with hemodynamically stable conditions. Critical care nurses are more likely to provide this comfort measure when the intervention (backrub) occurs immediately after the turn, because this approach saves time; the nurse does not have to remember to return in 5 to 15 minutes to give the backrub. Furthermore, the patient is disturbed only once. Generally speaking, it does not matter whether the patient is turned to the right side or the left side. However, if the patient is turned to the left, monitoring throughout the next 10 minutes would be prudent to confirm that SvO_2 returns to baseline levels. Nurses should also assess the other factors that influence SvO_2, including SaO_2, cardiac output, and hemoglobin level. Despite the generalizations suggested by our results, we strongly recommend that nurses initially evaluate each patient's response to intervention.

In conclusion, nurses must be cognizant that each nursing intervention affects the physiological status of the patient. Furthermore, combined interventions such as turning and backrub may affect the patient's hemodynamic state more dramatically than individual interventions do. In this era of managed care, it is important to consider both the most effective and the most cost-efficient manner of delivering interventions. Our data indicate that for postoperative cardiac patients with hemodynamically stable conditions, the standard practice of turning the patients and immediately giving a backrub is the best use of nursing time and causes little disruption of oxygen delivery or consumption.

ACKNOWLEDGMENTS
We thank Cheryl Scarmardo, Andreas Siskind, and Kimberly Buckley for their time and expertise in preparing the manuscript, figures, and graphs.

References

1. LUCKMAN J, SORENSEN KC, eds. *Medical-Surgical Nursing: A Psychophysiologic Approach.* Philadelphia, Pa: WB Saunders Co; 1993.

2. AHRENS T, RUTHERFORD K. *Essentials of Oxygenation.* Boston, Mass: Jones and Bartlett; 1993.

3. CERNAIANU AC, NELSON LD. The significance of mixed venous oxygen saturation and technical aspects of continuous measurement. In: Edwards JD, Shoemaker WC, Vincent JL, eds. *Oxygen Transport: Principles and Practices.* Philadelphia, Pa: WB Saunders Co; 1993: 99–124.

4. WHITE KM, WINSLOW EH, CLARK AP, TYLER DO. The physiologic basis for continuous mixed venous oxygen saturation monitoring. *Heart Lung.* 1990; 19:548–551.

5. SHIVELEY M. Effect of position change on mixed venous oxygen saturation in coronary artery bypass surgery patients. *Heart Lung.* 1988; 17:51–59.

6. TIDWELL, SL, RYAN WJ, OSGUTHORPE SG, PAULL DL, SMITH TL. Effect of position changes on mixed venous saturation in patients after coronary revascularization. *Heart Lung.* 1990: 19:574–578.

7. WINSLOW EH, CLARK AP, WHITE KM, TYLER DO. Effects of lateral turn on mixed venous oxygen saturation and heart rate in critically ill adults. *Heart Lung.* 1990; 19:557-566.

8. COPEL LC, STOLARIK A. Impact of nursing care activities on SvO_2 levels of postoperative cardiac surgery patients. *Cardiovasc Nurs.* 1991; 27:1–6.

9. ATKINS PJ, HAPSHE E, RIEGEL B. Effects of a bedbath on mixed venous oxygen saturation and heart rate in coronary artery bypass graft patients. *Am J Crit Care.* 1994; 3:107–115.

10. TYLER DO, WINSLOW EH, CLARK AP, WHITE KM. Effects of a 1-minute backrub on mixed venous oxygen saturation and heart rate in critically ill patients. *Heart Lung.* 1990; 19:562–565.

11. BARCIKOWSKI RS, ROBEY RR. Decisions in a single group repeated-measures analysis: statistical test and three computer packages. *Am Statistician.* 1984; 38:248–250.

12. BAELE PL, McMICHAN JC, MARSH HM, SILL JC, SOUTHORN PA. Continuous monitoring of mixed venous oxygen saturation in critically ill patients. *Anesth Analg.* 1982; 61:513–517.

13. WALLER JL, KAPLAN JA, BAUMAN DI, CRAVEN JM, Clinical evaluation of a new fiber-optic catheter oximeter during cardiac surgery. *Anesth Analg.* 1982; 61:676–679.

14. KROUSKOP RW, CABATU EE, CHELIAH BP, McDONNELL FE, BROWN EG. Accuracy and clinical utility of an oxygen saturation catheter. *Crit Care Med.* 1983; 11:744–749.

15. SHINNERS PA, PEASE MO. A stabilization period of 5 minutes is adequate when measuring pulmonary artery pressures after turning. *Am J Crit Care.* 1993; 2:474–477.

THE EFFECT OF A CORONARY ARTERY RISK EVALUATION PROGRAM ON SERUM LIPID VALUES AND CARDIOVASCULAR RISK LEVELS

SANDRA L. BRUCE AND SUSAN K. GROVE

In this study, serum lipid and cardiovascular risk levels of 195 military men and women were measured immediately before and 6 months after participation in a coronary artery risk evaluation (C.A.R.E.) program. Mean total cholesterol levels decreased from 257 mg/dl to 223 mg/dl ($t_{(194)}$ = –16.76, p = 0.00), low-density lipoprotein levels decreased from 170 mg/dl to 141 mg/dl ($t_{(194)}$ = –15.22, p = 0.00), and high-density lipoprotein levels increased from 45 mg/dl to 48 mg/dl ($t_{(194)}$ = 3.27, p = 0.01). Cardiovascular risk categories (based on serum lipid levels) were lowered from high to moderate risk in 54 subjects, high to low risk in 19 subjects, and moderate to low risk in 31 subjects (χ^2 = 98.28, p = 0.00). This study demonstrates that health education programs such as the C.A.R.E. Program can have a significant impact on serum lipid levels and cardiovascular risk levels and can potentially improve the health of high-risk populations.

Cardiovascular diseases cause nearly one of every two deaths in adults 45 years and older (American Heart Association, 1988). "It ranks first in terms of social security disability and second only to all forms of arthritis for limitation of activity, and to all forms of cancer combined for total hospital stays. In direct health care costs, lost wages, and productivity, coronary artery disease (CAD) costs the United States more than $60 billion a year" (Lipid Research Clinics [LRC] Program, p. 351).

Risk factors for CAD include male gender, family history of premature CAD, diabetes mellitus, hypertension, high cholesterol, cigarette smoking, and obesity (Expert Panel, 1988). The first three risk factors cannot be changed; however, the last four factors can be modified. Education can promote changes in daily living that reduce the risk for CAD (Glanz, 1988). The National Center for Health Statistics reports that slightly over 50% of Americans aged 20 to 74 have total blood cholesterol levels above the desirable level of 200 mg/dl. About 25% of the adult population is at high risk of CAD owing to levels of 240 mg/dl or greater and are candidates for intervention (Sempos, Fulwood, Hianes, & Cleeman, 1989).

Cholesterol is transported in the blood by lipoproteins. The low-density lipoprotein (LDL) carries most of the blood's cholesterol; high levels of LDL lead to atherosclerosis. The high-density lipoprotein (HDL) carries less of the blood cholesterol and helps prevent cholesterol deposition in the arteries (Kwiterovich, 1989). The goal of all risk-factor reduction strategies is to change blood lipid profiles from a "bad" one (high LDL, low HDL) to a "good" one (low LDL, high HDL). The purpose of this descriptive study was to compare a military population's mean levels of total serum cholesterol, LDL, HDL, and risk for cardiovascular disease (based on serum lipid levels) before and 6 months after a coronary artery risk evaluation (C.A.R.E.) program.

BACKGROUND

The Framingham study provided the first strong link between cholesterol, lipoproteins, and coronary artery disease in men and women (Kannel, Castelli, Gordon, & McNamara, 1971). Study results suggested that total serum cholesterol was the best indicator of CAD; people with elevated LDL cholesterol were more at risk than those with low levels of LDL. In addition, people with normal total cholesterol and low HDL cholesterol were more prone to cardiovascular disease than those with normal cholesterol and high HDL. For people at high risk for CAD, drugs were used to reduce their risk levels.

The LRC Coronary Primary Prevention Trial (1984) was a double-blind study that examined the effect of the lipid-lowering drug cholestyramine on the serum lipid levels and incidence of coronary events (number of heart attacks and deaths due to CAD) in approximately 4,000 men. Both the treatment group and the control group were placed on a low-saturated fat diet. Results from this trial demonstrated an 8.5% reduction in LDL cholesterol for the treatment group; this reduction was associated with a 19% reduction in CAD risk (LRC, 1984). These findings suggested that for every 1% reduction in blood cholesterol, CAD risk is reduced by 2% (National Institutes of Health [NIH], 1985).

The results of three clinical trials, the LRC Coronary Primary Prevention Trial (1984), The National Heart, Lung, and Blood Institute's Coronary Trial (NIH, 1985), and the Cholesterol-Lowering Atherosclerosis Study (Blankenhorn et al., 1987) found that an increase in HDL cholesterol produced a reduction in coronary artery disease in addition to the beneficial effect of lowering the LDL level (Kwiterovich, 1989). The Helsinki Heart Study was a rigorous experimental study on 4,081 asymptomatic, hypercholesterolemic men treated with a cholesterol-lowering diet or diet plus gemfibrozil (Fricke et al., 1987). Results demonstrated an 8% increase of HDL cholesterol and a 34% decrease in incidence of coronary events in the latter group. These results suggest that for every 1% increase in HDL level, there is about a 3% decrease in risk for CAD. This does not negate the additive effect of all risk factors in the development of CAD, but rather highlights the influence that serum LDL and HDL have in predicting risk (Cornett & Watson, 1984).

Nonpharmacological interventions also may be effective in reducing serum cholesterol. Peterson, Lefebvre, and Ferreira (1986) reported a 10.9% cholesterol reduction 6 months after intervention (one-time screening, counseling, health referrals, and follow-up screening), and

Quigley (1986) reported a 14% reduction in total cholesterol 8 months after intervention (screening, two 1-hour education sessions about cholesterol, and rescreening). The New York Telephone Company Trial reported a greater decrease in cholesterol (8.8%) in the treatment group (8-week education program that included nutrition education and training in self-management skills) than the control group (2.4%), as well as significantly greater weight loss (Bruno, Arnold, Jacobson, Winick, & Wynder, 1983). Each of these studies demonstrated positive effects from risk reduction education (Glanz, 1988).

Blair, Bryant, and Bocuzzi (1988) reported findings from an 18-month study conducted in a nurse-managed clinic for hyperlipidemic military personnel and their dependents. The subjects ($N = 86$) had cardiovascular disease and were treated with a cholesterol lowering diet and drugs. Thirty-two (37%) of the subjects were able to lower their mean cholesterol from 299 mg/dl to 241 mg/dl (19% reduction) on dietary therapy alone, and 54 (63%) achieved a 25% decrease in mean cholesterol from 310 mg/dl to 231 mg/dl on diet and drug therapy. This study highlighted the effectiveness of nursing interventions in individuals with hyperlipidemia.

In March 1988, the Strategic Air Command Surgeon General directed medical facilities to provide a means for military members to voluntarily obtain information regarding their lipid status and risk for cardiovascular disease. The staff of an outpatient primary care clinic in Texas developed the C.A.R.E. program to effect positive health outcomes (reduction in CAD risk) through a lipid screening and education intervention. This study evaluated the relationship between an education intervention (the C.A.R.E. program) and health outcomes (decreased serum lipids and cardiovascular risk). The following research question was developed for the study: What is the difference in the mean total serum cholesterol, LDL cholesterol, and HDL cholesterol and cardiovascular risk levels of military members before and after participation in the C.A.R.E. program?

METHOD

Sample: The setting was the outpatient primary care clinic of a 140-bed military hospital that serves men and women who are active duty or retired from active duty as well as their dependents over the age of 16 years. The C.A.R.E. program was advertised in the clinic lobby and the base newspaper as a service for anyone interested in learning about their lipid levels and risk of heart disease. Although it was mandated by the Strategic Air Command Surgeon General to provide this service, participation was voluntary.

The Expert Panel of the National Heart, Lung, and Blood Institute's National Cholesterol Education Program (NCEP) has established guidelines for detecting, evaluating, and treating hypercholesterolemia. These guidelines formed the standards for the intervention used in this study (Figure 1). As a result of the growing understanding about the role of cholesterol in CAD, the NCEP was developed to inform health professionals and the public about the importance of monitoring serum cholesterol levels (Expert Panel, 1988).

**Figure 1. C.A.R.E. guidelines adapted from the NCEP.
(Reprinted from Expert Panel, 1988.)**

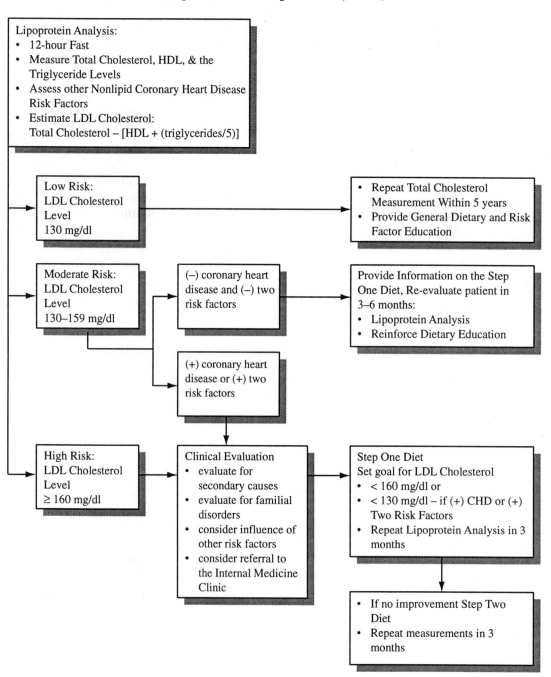

The C.A.R.E. program was conducted for a period of one year, and a total of 483 individuals were voluntarily screened. Fifteen of these individuals were referred immediately to the internal medicine clinic because of dangerously high lipid values (serum cholesterol greater than 300 mg/dl) and two or more nonlipid risk factors. These individuals were not included in the study sample. Those with cholesterol values less than 200 mg/dl (and the absence of other nonlipid risk factors) were considered low risk. Owing to their low risk, these individuals (*n* = 122) were instructed to have follow-up blood levels drawn in one year and were not included in the sample. One hundred twenty-seven individuals did not return for follow-up evaluation and were not included in the study sample. Twenty-four of the individuals screened did not meet the following sample criteria: (a) greater than 16 years of age; (b) military members (active duty, retired, or dependent); (c) not under pharmacological treatment for hyperlipidemia; (d) English-speaking; (e) triglycerides under 400 mg/dl (this criterion was set because the calculation for LDL is not accurate for individuals for triglyceride values greater than 400 mg/dl); (f) nondiabetic; and (g) no current referrals to other health providers. Of the 483 individuals screened, 195 became research subjects. A power analysis was performed to confirm the adequacy of the sample size (Cohen, 1988).

The sample consisted of 92 men and 103 women and included 36 married couples. The subjects ranged from 20 to 80 years of age, with a mean age of 53.33 years (± 13 SD). Information about the subjects' body mass index (BMI), systolic blood pressure (SBP), diastolic blood pressure (DBP), heart rate, and glucose are provided in Table 1. The means for these variables were within normal limits.

Procedure: The data (serum lipid values and individual risk factor information) were obtained through retrospective medical record review and coded in order to protect the subject's identity. Measurements of the total serum cholesterol, the HDL, the LDL, and the estimated cardiovascular risk level were compared before and 6 months after participation in the program. The

Table 1. Means, standard deviations, and ranges of the physiological attributes of the sample (92 men and 103 women).

ATTRIBUTE	$\bar{x}$	SD	RANGE
[a]BMI (Kg/cm^2)	25.03	2.82	19.57–37.19
SBP (mmHg)	135.08	17.72	100–178
DBP (mmHg)	82.98	8.51	54–102
Heart Rate	85.33	8.11	64–104
Serum Glucose (mg/dl)	97.83	13.83	72–130

Abbreviations: SBP, systolic blood pressure; DBP, diastolic blood pressure; BMI, body mass index, [a]BMI: 19 = lean; 25 = average; 31 = heavy (Kwiterovich, 1989).

C.A.R.E. program was a voluntary program that offered screening, evaluation, and cardiac risk reduction education to all eligible military personnel. Screening consisted of an interview by the nurse manager of the program to determine individual risk factors and to provide instructions for obtaining a fasting lipid profile and glucose. The participants also had their height, weight, and blood pressure checked. Each person then was enrolled in the next available C.A.R.E. class.

In the evaluation phase, the program nurse, in conjunction with the clinic physician, assessed the person's cardiac risk status based on reported risk factors and the results of the serum lipid profile, according to NCEP guidelines. Each C.A.R.E. participant was determined to have low, moderate, or high risk for cardiovascular disease. Recommendations were made based on this risk classification and individual considerations. These recommendations included dietary guidelines, exercise guidelines, follow-up instructions, and in some cases, formal referrals to other resources.

The educational phase of the program involved attending a C.A.R.E. class. This 90-minute class provided instruction concerning cardiovascular health, emphasizing the relationship between daily living behaviors, and identification of risk factors that determine one's risk for heart disease. At the beginning of this group session, each participant was given a handout that included the following information: their serum lipid profile results; their risk classification (high, moderate, or low); and specific individualized recommendations. The results of the lipid profiles and risk-level evaluations were explained in detail. Dietary instruction on the Step-One Diet (Table 2) was provided, as recommended by the Expert Panel (1988). Copies of the Step-One Diet were given to each person. General behavioral changes were recommended to the participants, such as reducing sedentary behaviors and maintaining ideal body weight. At

Table 2. Dietary guidelines to lower blood cholesterol.

	RECOMMENDED INTAKE	
NUTRIENT	STEP-ONE DIET	STEP-TWO DIET
Total Fat	<30% of total calories	<30% of total calories
Saturated fatty acids	<10% of total calories	<7% of total calories
Polyunsaturated fatty acids	0% to 10% of total calories	0% to 10% of total calories
Carbohydrates	10% to 15% of total calories	10% to 15% of total calories
Protein	50% to 60% of total calories	50% to 60% of total calories
Cholesterol	10% to 20% of total calories	10% to 20% of total calories
	<300 mg/day	<200 mg/day
	To achieve and maintain desirable weight	To achieve and maintain desirable weight

Reprinted from Expert Panel (1998).

the close of the class, recommendations and follow-up instructions were discussed with each participant individually. The subjects also received follow-up screening and counseling (based on rescreening results) 6 months after the start of the program.

Measures: A standardized protocol for lipid data collection, prescribed by the NCEP, was followed by each subject: (a) fast for 12 hours; (b) maintain stable dietary patterns for at least three weeks; (c) maintain stable body weight; (d) be neither ill nor pregnant; and (e) have no recent history of myocardial infarction, less than 3 months. The laboratory values of total serum, LDL, and HDL cholesterol from this agency met the referenced criteria ($\pm$ 3% of the true value) set by the NCEP. The true value is an accepted reference value, established by the National Bureau of Standards (NBS) or the Centers for Disease Control (Finney, 1990). The level of LDL cholesterol was calculated using the following equation developed by Friedewald, Levy, and Fredrickson (1972): Total cholesterol – [HDL cholesterol + (triglycerides/5)] = LDL.

RESULTS

The most prevalent nonlipid risk factor present for this sample was a family history of coronary artery disease; 73 (37.4%) of the subjects reported that definite myocardial infarction or sudden death had occurred before the age of 65 years in a parent or sibling. Incidence of other reported risk factors were as follows: cigarette smoking, 22.1%; hypertension (SBP 140 mmHg; DBP 90 mmHg), 15.9%; obesity (greater than or equal to 30% over ideal body weight), 5.6%; and diagnosed coronary artery disease, 3.1%.

Six months after participation in the C.A.R.E. program, the mean total cholesterol was reduced by 33.82 mg/dl ($t(194) = -16.76$, $p = 0.00$), and the mean LDL level was reduced by 28.97 mg/dl ($t(194) = -15.22$, $p = 0.00$). The mean HDL cholesterol was increased by 2.75 mg/dl ($t(194) = 3.27$, $p = 0.001$) (Table 3).

Table 3. Baseline and follow-up mean cholesterol levels (mg/dl) in study population (92 men and 103 women).

TYPE OF CHOLESTEROL	BASELINE		FOLLOW-UP			
	$\bar{x}$	SD	$\bar{x}$	SD	*t* VALUE	*p*
Total serum cholesterol	257.20	36.43	223.38	34.05	–16.75	0.0000
LDL cholesterol	170.40	36.52	141.43	32.24	–15.22	0.0000
HDL cholesterol	44.83	15.01	47.58	13.00	+3.27	0.0012

Abbreviations: LDL, low-density lipoprotein; HDL, high-density lipoprotein.

**Figure 2. Percentage of subjects in each cardiovascular risk category
before and after treatment (*P* = .0000).**

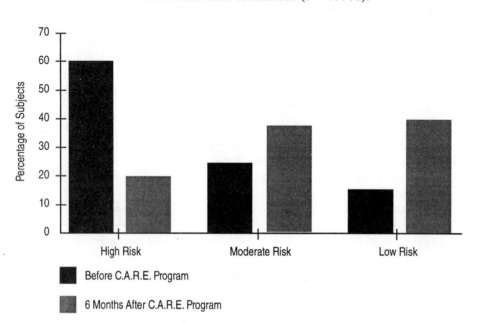

The risk levels of the subjects before and 6 months after the C.A.R.E. program were compared. Using a 3 × 3 – chi-square table, the sample was categorized into low, moderate, and
high risk for cardiovascular disease based on the serum lipid profile and nonlipid risk factors
before and after participation (Figure 2). The number of subjects in the high-risk category
before participation was 116 (59.5%) and was reduced to 45 (23.1%) after participation; 50
(25.6%) were in the moderate-risk category before participation and 71 (36.4%) after participation; and 29 (14.9%) were in the low-risk category before participation and 79 (40.5%) after
participation. The increased number of subjects in the moderate-risk group after participation
is accounted for by the movement of high-risk individuals to the moderate-risk category. Cardiovascular risk categories were lowered from high to moderate risk in 54 subjects; high to low
risk in 19 subjects; and moderate to low risk in 31 subjects; 43 remained high risk; 17 remained
moderate risk; and 29 remained in low risk. Only two individuals went from moderate to high
risk. Significant changes in risk factor categorization were noted using an extension of the
McNemar Test for Significance of Changes (Bowker, 1948; McNemar, 1947). The value obtained (χ^2 greater than 98.285, p = 0.00) was 12.6 times larger than the critical value of χ^2 =
7.815 (0.95, df = 3), demonstrating a significant difference in the cardiovascular risk levels of
the group posttreatment.

DISCUSSION

The screening process was beneficial in identifying individuals with health risks. Fifteen individuals were referred for medical intervention because of dangerously high cardiovascular risk levels. Eleven other subjects were referred for evaluation of hypertension, and 6 subjects were referred for elevated fasting serum glucose levels.

As expected, strong correlations were found between cardiovascular risk and the total cholesterol level ($r = .67$, $p = .000$; 44% variance explained) and the LDL cholesterol level ($r = .80$, $p = .000$; 64% variance explained). However, HDL cholesterol did not correlate significantly with cardiovascular risk level ($r = -.12$; 1.5% of the variance explained), which is unexpected because the literature supports this correlation (Lipid Research Clinics Program, 1984; Fricke et al., 1987; Levy et al., 1984; Pocock, Shaper, & Phillips, 1989).

A significant 13% decrease in the mean total serum cholesterol level occurred after participation in the C.A.R.E. program. Based on the premise that a 1% reduction in serum cholesterol produces a 2% reduction in cardiovascular risk, the participants in this study could have achieved an overall 26% reduction in risk for coronary heart disease (LRC, 1984; NIH, 1985). Several nonpharmacological cardiovascular education intervention studies reported similar reductions in total serum cholesterol levels. Peterson and colleagues (1986) reported a 11% mean reduction of total cholesterol 6 months after interventions; Quigley (1986) reported a 14% reduction in total cholesterol levels 8 months after an education program; and Bruno and colleagues (1983) reported a 9% reduction 6 months after intervention. Thus, the 13% reduction in total serum cholesterol after the C.A.R.E. program was consistent with other nonpharmacological education interventions.

Mean LDL levels decreased 17% after participation in the C.A.R.E. program. A LDL level greater than 160 mg/dl constitutes high risk for cardiovascular disease regardless of the presence of other risk factors. The participants in the C.A.R.E. program reduced their mean LDL level from 170.40 to 140.43 mg/dl (17% reduction) and on the basis of this factor alone lowered their overall risk classification from high to moderate.

Mean HDL cholesterol level increased 5.8% after participation in the C.A.R.E. program. Results from the Helsinki Heart Study suggest that for every 1% increase in HDL level, a 3% decrease in risk for CAD occurs (Fricke et al., 1987). According to this premise, the study subjects decreased their risk for coronary heart disease by 17.4%.

The majority (99.5%) of the subjects either decreased their cardiovascular risk classification or remained in the same classification after participation in the C.A.R.E. program. Only 2 (1%) of the 195 participants increased their risk levels (from moderate to high risk). This could be attributed to noncompliance to the C.A.R.E. program guidelines or familial hyperlipidemia (Kwiterovich, 1989). The latter may require pharmacological intervention. Overall, positive changes in the participants' blood lipid levels and cardiovascular risk classification were noted after participation in the C.A.R.E. program.

Several factors must be considered when interpreting these findings. In this descriptive study, the original risk was based on the serum lipid profile and the presence of nonlipid risk factors as indicated by the Expert Panel (1988), and the changes in risk classification are based on changes in the lipid values only. Other variables known to affect cardiovascular risk (e.g., exercise, smoking, hypertension, body weight) were not reexamined after participation in the C.A.R.E. program. There may have been an even greater magnitude of change in risk classification if other risk factors were measured postparticipation. "Regression toward the mean" may have been responsible for some of the cholesterol reduction because single determinations were used to establish baseline and end-of-participation blood lipid levels (Green & Lewis, 1986). The findings may demonstrate an association between the C.A.R.E. program and the improvements in serum lipid values for the sample. However, quasi-experimental studies with control groups are needed to examine the full impact of the program.

Because the study was limited to 6 months after participation in the C.A.R.E. program, long-term trends were not examined. Future research should include longitudinal studies to assess the degree to which behavior changes are sustained over time. Examining different populations such as minorities, women, children, and the elderly would strengthen the findings. Finally, a cost-benefit analysis could highlight potential savings in terms of health-care costs for high-risk individuals.

Health education has long been an integral component of professional nursing. Indeed, nurses can be viewed as a primary source of health information. Education does not have to be lengthy to be beneficial. The simple changes corresponding to those of the NCEP's Step-One Diet can be recommended by a nurse in a few minutes. The results do support the use of educational programs in addition to risk factor assessment in reducing cardiac risk levels. Education can be effective in improving lipid profiles and potentially decrease the incidence of CAD. Decreasing risk for CAD and the associated loss of productivity, disability, and death could enhance quality of life. This study demonstrates that nurse-managed health education programs such as the C.A.R.E. program can have dramatic impact on individuals' health and can potentially improve quality of life for high-risk populations.

From the Sheppard Air Force Base, and the University of Texas at Arlington, TX.

SANDRA L. BRUCE, MSN, RN, CCRN: Major, United States Air Force, Nurse Corps. Sheppard Air Force Base, TX; SUSAN K. GROVE, PhD, RN: Professor, Assistant Dean, The University of Texas at Arlington School of Nursing.

Address reprint requests to Sandra L. Bruce, MSN, RN, CCRN, Major, United States Air Force, 383d Medical Training Squadron/NTOE, 939 Missile Rd., Suite 3, Sheppard Air Force Base, TX, 76311-2262.

0897-1897/94/0702-0004$0.00/0

References

AMERICAN HEART ASSOCIATION (1988). *Recommendations for treatment of hyperlipidemia in adults.* Dallas, TX: American Heart Association.

BLAIR, T.P., BRYANT, J., & BOCUZZI, S. (1988). Treatment of hypercholesterolemia by a clinical nurse using a stepped-care protocol in a nonvolunteer population. *Archives of Internal Medicine, 148,* 1046–1048.

BLANKENHORN, D.H., NESSIM, S.A., JOHNSON, R.L., SAN MARCO, M.E., AZEN, A.P., & CASHEN-HEMPHILL, L. (1987). Beneficial effects of combined colestipol-niacin therapy on coronary atherosclerosis and coronary artery vs bypass grafts. *JAMA, 257,* 3233–3240.

BOWKER, A.H. (1948). A test for symmetry in contingency tables. *Journal of the American Statistical Association, 43,* 572–574.

BRUNO, R., ARNOLD, C., JACOBSON, L., WINICK, M., & WYNDER, E. (1983). Randomized trial of a nonpharmacologic cholesterol reduction program at the worksite. *Preventive Medicine, 12,* 523–532.

COHEN, J. (1988). *Statistical power analysis for the behavioral sciences* (2nd ed.). Hillsdale, NJ: Lawrence and Earlbam Associates.

EXPERT PANEL (1988). *Report of the National Cholesterol Education Program Expert Panel on detection, evaluation, and treatment of high blood cholesterol in adults* (US Dept of Health and Human Resources Publication No. NIH 88-2925.) Washington, DC: National Heart, Lung, and Blood Institute.

FINNEY, C.P. (1990). Measurement issues in cholesterol screening: An overview for nurses. *Journal of Cardiovascular Nursing, 5*(2), 10–22.

FRIEDEWALD, W.T., LEVY, R.I., & FREDRICKSON, D.S. (1972). Estimation of the concentration of low-density lipoprotein cholesterol in plasma, without the use of the preparative ultracentrifuge. *Clinical Chemistry, 18,* 499–502.

FRICKE, M.H., ELO, O., HAAPA, K., HEINONEN, O.P., HEINSALMI, P., HELO, P., HUTTUNEN, J.K., KAITANIEMI, P., KOSKINEN, P., MANNINEN, V., MAENPAA, H., MALKONEN, M., MANTTARI, M., NOVOLA, S., PATERNICK, A., PIKKARAINEN, J., ROMO, M., SJOBLOM, T., & NIKKILA, E.A. (1987). Helsinki heart study: Primary prevention trial with gemfibrozil in middle-aged men with dyslipidemia. *New England Journal of Medicine, 317,* 1237–1245.

GLANZ, K. (1988). Patient and public education for cholesterol reduction: A review of strategies and issues. *Patient Education and Counseling, 12,* 235–257.

GREEN, L.W., KREUTER, M.W., DEEDS, S.G., & PARTRIDGE, K.B. (1980). *Health education and planning: A diagnostic approach.* Palo Alto, CA: Mayfield.

GREEN, L.W., & LEWIS, F.M. (1986). *Measurement and evaluation in health education and promotion.* Palo Alto, CA: Mayfield.

KANNEL, W.B., CASTELLI, W.P., GORDON, T., & MCNAMARA, P.M. (1971). Serum cholesterol, lipoproteins, and the risk of coronary heart disease: The Framingham study. *Annals of Internal Medicine, 74,* 1–12.

KWITEROVICH, P. (1989). *Beyond cholesterol: The Johns Hopkins complete guide for avoiding heart disease.* Baltimore, MD: Johns Hopkins University Press.

LEVY, R.F., BRENSIKE, J.F., EPSTEIN, S.E., KELSEY, S.F., PASSAMANI, E.R., RICHARDSON, J.W., LOH, I.K., STONE, N.I., ALDRICH, R.F., BATTAGLINI, J.W., MORIARTY, D.J., FISHER, M.L., FRIEDMAN, L., FRIEDEWALD, W., & DETRE, K.M. (1984). The influence of changes in lipid values induced by cholestyramine and diet on progression of coronary artery disease results of the NHLBI, type II coronary intervention study. *Circulation, 69,* 325–327.

LIPID RESEARCH CLINICS PROGRAM (1984). The lipid research clinics coronary primary prevention trial results I. Reduction in incidence of coronary heart disease to cholesterol lowering. *JAMA, 251,* 351–364.

McNEMAR, Q. (1947). Note on the sampling error of the difference between correlated proportions of percentages. *Psychometrika, 12,* 153–157.

NATIONAL INSTITUTES OF HEALTH (1985). Consensus development conference statement: Lowering blood cholesterol to prevent heart disease. *JAMA, 253,* 2080–2086.

PETERSON, G.S., LEFEBVRE, R.C., & FERREIRA, A. (1968). Strategies for cholesterol lowering at the worksite. *Journal of Nutrition Education, 18*(2), S54–S57.

POCOCK, S.J., SHAPER, A.G., & PHILLIPS, A.N. (1989). Concentrations of high density lipoprotein cholesterol, triglycerides, and total cholesterol in ischemic heart disease. *The British Journal of Medicine, 72,* 998–1002.

QUIGLEY, H.L. (1986). L.L. Bean cholesterol reduction program. *Journal of Nutrition Education, 18*(2) S58–S59.

SEMPOS, C., FULWOOD, R., HAINES, C., & CLEEMAN, J. (1989). The prevalence of high blood cholesterol levels among adults in the United States. *JAMA, 262,* 45–51.

Reprinted from Applied Nursing Research, *Vol. 7, No. 2 (May).*